Department of Veterans Affairs
Health Services Research & Development Service | Evidence-based Synthesis Program

HSR&D

Nutritional Supplements for Age-related Macular Degeneration: A Systematic Review

January 2012

Prepared for:
Department of Veterans Affairs
Veterans Health Administration
Health Services Research & Development Service
Washington, DC 20420

Prepared by:
Evidence-based Synthesis Program (ESP) Center
Portland VA Medical Center
Portland, OR
Devan Kansagara, MD, MCR, Director

Investigators:
Principal Investigator:
Devan Kansagara, MD, MCR

Co-Investigators:
Ken Gleitsmann, MD, MPH
Melanie Gillingham, PhD, RD
Michele Freeman, MPH
Ana Quiñones, PhD

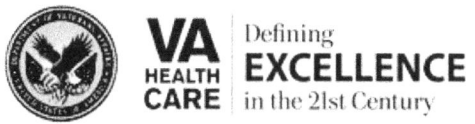

VA
HEALTH
CARE | Defining
EXCELLENCE
in the 21st Century

PREFACE

Health Services Research & Development Service's (HSR&D's) Evidence-based Synthesis Program (ESP) was established to provide timely and accurate syntheses of targeted healthcare topics of particular importance to Veterans Affairs (VA) managers and policymakers, as they work to improve the health and healthcare of Veterans. The ESP disseminates these reports throughout VA.

HSR&D provides funding for four ESP Centers and each Center has an active VA affiliation. The ESP Centers generate evidence syntheses on important clinical practice topics, and these reports help:

- develop clinical policies informed by evidence,
- guide the implementation of effective services to improve patient outcomes and to support VA clinical practice guidelines and performance measures, and
- set the direction for future research to address gaps in clinical knowledge.

In 2009, the ESP Coordinating Center was created to expand the capacity of HSR&D Central Office and the four ESP sites by developing and maintaining program processes. In addition, the Center established a Steering Committee comprised of HSR&D field-based investigators, VA Patient Care Services, Office of Quality and Performance, and Veterans Integrated Service Networks (VISN) Clinical Management Officers. The Steering Committee provides program oversight, guides strategic planning, coordinates dissemination activities, and develops collaborations with VA leadership to identify new ESP topics of importance to Veterans and the VA healthcare system.

Comments on this evidence report are welcome and can be sent to Nicole Floyd, ESP Coordinating Center Program Manager, at nicole.floyd@va.gov.

Recommended citation: Kansagara D, Gleitsmann K, Gillingham M, Freeman M, Quiñones A. Nutritional Supplements for Age-related Macular Degeneration: A Systematic Review. VA-ESP Project #05-225; 2011

This report is based on research conducted by the Evidence-based Synthesis Program (ESP) Center located at the Portland VA Medical Center, Portland OR funded by the Department of Veterans Affairs, Veterans Health Administration, Office of Research and Development, Health Services Research and Development. The findings and conclusions in this document are those of the author(s) who are responsible for its contents; the findings and conclusions do not necessarily represent the views of the Department of Veterans Affairs or the United States government. Therefore, no statement in this article should be construed as an official position of the Department of Veterans Affairs. No investigators have any affiliations or financial involvement (e.g., employment, consultancies, honoraria, stock ownership or options, expert testimony, grants or patents received or pending, or royalties) that conflict with material presented in the report.

TABLE OF CONTENTS

EXECUTIVE SUMMARY

BACKGROUND

Age-related macular degeneration (AMD) is the leading cause of irreversible vision loss in the developed world. In 2004, AMD affected 1.75 million persons in the United States, a number that is expected to rise to nearly 3 million by 2020 due to the aging of the population.

The severity of macular degeneration ranges from Category 1 (least severe) to Category 4 (most severe), and "advanced AMD" is defined as having geographic atrophy involving the center of the macula or features of choroidal neovascularization.

Observational studies suggest that people with dietary intakes higher in various carotenoids, antioxidants and omega-3 fatty acids have a lower risk of developing AMD. This has led to several supplementation trials designed to examine the ability of nutritional supplement with carotenoids, antioxidants, or omega-3 fatty acids to prevent the progression of AMD.

Our report focuses on the evidence documenting the potential benefits and harms of certain dietary supplements in patients with AMD. We conducted a systematic review of published literature to address the following key questions:

1) In patients with age-related macular degeneration, do nutritional supplements containing carotenoids, antioxidants, or omega-3 fatty acids alone or in combination prevent functional visual loss?

2) In adult populations, what are the harms of carotenoid, antioxidant, and omega-3 fatty acid supplementation?

METHODS

We conducted searches in Medline® Embase, Scopus, Conference Papers Index, and the Cochrane Library (Cochrane Database of Systematic Reviews; Database of Abstracts of Reviews of Effects; Cochrane Central Register of Controlled Trials) from 1947 or database inception through February 2011. We obtained additional articles from systematic reviews, reference lists of pertinent studies, reviews, editorials, and by consulting experts. Reviewers trained in the critical analysis of literature assessed for relevance the abstracts of citations identified from literature searches. Full-text articles of potentially relevant abstracts were retrieved for further review. We assessed the internal validity of each study using the Cochrane Risk of Bias tool. We assessed the overall quality of the body of evidence for each outcome by considering the consistency, coherence, and applicability across studies, as well as the internal validity of individual studies, using a method developed by the Grades of Recommendation, Assessment, Development, and Evaluation (GRADE) Working Group. We critically analyzed the evidence on efficacy and adverse effects, and compiled a narrative synthesis of findings.

RESULTS

We reviewed 4,335 titles and abstracts from the electronic search, and identified 22 additional references through manual searching of reference lists or from input from technical advisors.

After applying inclusion/exclusion criteria at the abstract level, 347 full-text articles were reviewed. Of the full-text articles, we rejected 308 that did not meet our inclusion criteria.

Key Question #1. In patients with age-related macular degeneration, do nutritional supplements containing carotenoids, antioxidants, or omega-3 fatty acids alone or in combination prevent functional visual loss?

We identified seven randomized controlled trials (RCTs) of nutritional supplements in AMD patients. A significant effect in preventing functional loss was found only in the two largest trials. The weight of evidence was dominated by the Age Related Eye Disease Study (AREDS) in terms of sample size (N=3640) and duration of follow-up (7 years). The sample sizes in the other six studies ranged from 60 to 164 subjects, with follow-up ranging from 6 to 24 months. Given that progression of AMD occurs slowly and with low frequency, the smaller studies might have been of insufficient duration or power to detect a treatment effect.

In the AREDS study, a beneficial effect was observed with a combination of antioxidants (500 mg vitamin C, 400 IU vitamin E, and 15 mg beta carotene) plus zinc (80 mg zinc oxide and 2 mg cupric oxide) but only among subjects with Categories 3 and 4 AMD. No significant change was reported in mild AMD subjects (Category 1 or 2) in any of the three treatment arms (i.e., antioxidants alone; zinc alone; or antioxidants plus zinc) compared with placebo. The protective effect of greatest magnitude among all of the supplement treatment arms was noted in the zinc plus antioxidant group (OR 0.63, 99% CI 0.44-0.92).

Key Question #2. In adult populations, what are the harms of carotenoid, antioxidant, and omega-3 fatty acid supplementation?

Vitamin E at high doses (>=400 IU/day) may be associated with increased risk of mortality, congestive heart failure, and prostate cancer.

Beta-carotene may be associated with an increased risk of lung cancer among active smokers. In the Beta-Carotene and Retinol Efficacy Trial (CARET) and Alpha-Tocopherol and Beta-Carotene (ATBC) trials, beta-carotene was associated with increased mortality and increased risk of lung cancer among smokers. Two other large trials, the Women's Health Study (WHS) and the Physicians' Health Study (PHS), did not find an excess risk of lung cancer among smokers using beta-carotene, but a meta-analysis combining these four studies determined that the overall risk of lung cancer among current smokers treated with beta-carotene was significantly elevated (OR 1.24 (95% CI, 1.10-1.39)). No increase in lung cancer incidence was observed among former smokers and nonsmokers in these studies. In prospective cohort studies that used lower doses than RCTs, a small inverse association between carotenoids and lung cancer among current smokers has been observed.

Zinc was associated with urinary tract infections and hospital admissions due to genitourinary causes in one study.

Yellowish discoloration of the skin was frequently reported in trials of beta-carotene, and has also been noted in trials of lutein. Gastrointestinal symptoms were also commonly reported in trials of various supplements.

DISCUSSION

We found good evidence mainly from one large RCT (AREDS) that supplementation with carotenoids and antioxidants decreased the risk of functional vision loss among patients with Category 3 or 4 AMD. One smaller RCT also found zinc supplementation may decrease the risk of clinically significant visual loss among patients with Category 3 or 4 AMD. The effects of carotenoids or omega-3 fatty acids alone have not been well-studied. An ongoing study (AREDS II) is currently being conducted to evaluate the effects of carotenoids (lutein and zeaxanthin) and omega-3 fatty acids (DHA and EPA) on AMD progression in approximately 4,200 subjects with Categories 3 to 4 AMD.

In the AREDS trial, there was no detectable effect on vision loss in any of the treatment arms among subjects with Category 1 or 2 AMD, due to the very slow rate of disease progression in these subjects. Based on the findings of AREDS, we estimate that a trial of Category 2 AMD patients would need an approximate sample size of 17,000 subjects, followed for at least five years, to detect a significant difference in functional vision loss associated with supplementation.

Higher doses of vitamin E (>400 IU per day) have been associated with an estimated four percent increase in mortality; a 13 to 17 percent increase in risk of prostate cancer; and a 13 to 50 percent increase in risk of congestive heart failure among those with existing CVD risk factors such as left ventricular dysfunction, diabetes mellitus, recent myocardial infarction, or renal insufficiency. Carotenoids such as beta-carotene have been associated with an estimated 24 percent increase in risk of lung cancer among smokers. Whether the balance of benefits and harms favors supplementation in AMD patients likely depends on the population being considered. There is strong evidence for benefit in patients with more advanced AMD, and in these patients, the very small risk of harm is likely to be outweighed by the potential benefit.

CONCLUSION

Evidence of benefit from supplementation with carotenoids and antioxidants on functional vision loss in patients with AMD is based mainly on the results of one large trial. The observed benefit occurred only among subjects with Category 3 or 4 AMD. There is evidence for a low risk of harm from some nutritional supplements at high doses. As with any clinical intervention, the balance of benefits and harms regarding supplementation in AMD patients depends on the population being considered. Given that AMD patients are older and have additional medical comorbidities, many would be at risk for some of the potential harms associated with supplementation. The precautionary principle should be observed while further evidence evolves.

While our report notes the uncertainty in the conclusions of many of the included studies, reasonable recommendations can be extended:

- Carotenoid and antioxidant supplements significantly decrease visual loss and can be recommended for patients with Categories 3 and 4 AMD.
- Current literature does not support the use of these supplements for patients with mild AMD.
- Certain nutritional supplements have significant potential harms:
    - Increased mortality and congestive heart failure in high risk patients with vitamin E.
    - Increased risk of prostate cancer with vitamin E.
    - Increased risk of lung cancer among smokers with beta-carotene.

The table below summarizes the evidence on the benefits and harms of oral supplements for AMD.

EXECUTIVE SUMMARY TABLE

Summary of the evidence of the effects of nutritional supplements in patients with age-related macular degeneration

Outcome	Treatment	Population	Effect*	GRADE Classification†	Comment
Functional vision loss	Carotenoids	Early AMD	(~)	Low	Single study (N=90) found a small increase in visual acuity after 12 months, but the improvement was not clinically significant (i.e. <15 letters).
	Antioxidants‡	Categories 3-4 AMD	(+)	Moderate	Evidence of benefit from 1 large multicenter trial (AREDS) and 1 smaller trial. 4 small trials found neutral effects on functional vision loss.
	Antioxidants	Category 2 AMD	(~)	Low	No evidence of benefit after 7 years of treatment in 1 large multicenter trial (AREDS) that included 1,063 Category 2 subjects.
	Omega-3 fatty acids	Early AMD (94% in Categories 1-2)	(~)	Very low	1 study found evidence of slowed visual acuity loss but not to a clinically significant degree. Very few subjects in this study (6.4%) had Categories 3-4 AMD.
Quality of life	Carotenoids	AMD	(~)	Low	No significant findings on night driving in one study (N=90).
	Antioxidants	N/A	(0)	N/A	No evidence.
	Omega-3 fatty acids	N/A	(0)	N/A	No evidence.
Mortality	Beta-carotene	Smokers	(−)	Moderate	High-dose beta-carotene (20 to 30 mg/day) was linked with increased mortality in 2 large trials in smokers and asbestos workers.
	Vitamin E	General population	(−)	High	High-dose vitamin E (>=400 IU/day) was associated with a slight increase in mortality in a meta-analysis of 11 trials.
Lung cancer	Beta-carotene	Smokers	(−)	Moderate	High-dose beta-carotene (20 to 30 mg/day) was linked with increased lung cancer incidence among smokers in a meta-analysis of 4 large trials. No increase in lung cancer was observed among former and non-smokers.
Prostate cancer	Vitamin E	General population	(−)	Low	High-dose vitamin E (400 IU/day) was associated with an increase in prostate cancer in one study.
Gastrointestinal cancers	Antioxidants	General population	(~)	High	Supplements had no effect on incidence of gastrointestinal cancers in a meta-analysis of 12 good-quality trials.

**Nutritional Supplements for Age-related Macular Degeneration:
A Systematic Review**

Outcome	Treatment	Population	Effect*	GRADE Classification†	Comment
Congestive heart failure	Vitamin E	DM, CVD, or post-infarction	(–)	Low	Vitamin E (300-400 IU/day) was linked with increased CHF hospitalization in 2 trials of high-risk patients.
Urinary tract infections (UTIs)	Zinc	AMD	(–)	Low	Zinc (80 mg/day) was associated with more UTIs and hospital admissions due to genitourinary causes compared with non-zinc treated subjects in one large study.
Yellowing of the skin	Beta-carotene Lutein	AMD and general population	(–)	High	Transient yellowing of the skin was frequently reported in trials of beta-carotene and in two trials of lutein.
Gastrointestinal (GI) symptoms	Antioxidants	AMD	(–)	High	GI symptoms were the most common adverse effect that led to withdrawal from studies, according to a systematic review of 10 RCTs of antioxidant supplements for AMD.

GRADE = Grades of Recommendation, Assessment, Development, and Evaluation; ICU = intensive care unit; RCT = randomized controlled trial; AMD = age-related macular degeneration; CHF = congestive heart failure.

* Effect: (+) benefit; (–) harm; (~) mixed findings/no effect; (0) no evidence.

† GRADE classification: high = further research is very unlikely to change our confidence on the estimate of effect; moderate = further research is likely to have an important impact on our confidence in the estimate of effect and may change the estimate; low = further research is very likely to have an important impact on our confidence in the estimate of effect and is likely to change the estimate; very low = any estimate of effect is very uncertain.

‡ Trials of antioxidants included treatment with antioxidants alone or combined with carotenoids or other supplements.

EVIDENCE REPORT

INTRODUCTION

Age-related macular degeneration (AMD) is the leading cause of irreversible vision loss in the developed world. In 2004, AMD affected 1.75 million persons in the United States, a number which is expected to rise to nearly 3 million by 2020 due to the aging of the population.[1] AMD is characterized by the appearance of involutional changes (e.g. drusen) in the structure of the central retinal pigment epithelium (RPE) leading to the loss of normal central (macular) vision. AMD can be categorized as dry (non-exudative) or wet (exudative). Dry AMD represents the great majority of AMD patients (90%) and may lead to slow visual loss over many decades, with the most severe cases developing geographic atrophy and profound loss of central vision. Dry AMD can progress to wet AMD with the development of neovascularization beneath the diseased RPE leading to hemorrhage, scarring, and the devastating loss of macular vision over a period of months.

By convention, there are four categories which describe the severity of macular degeneration. Category 1 are those patients essentially free of age-related macular abnormalities, with a total drusen area less than five small drusen (63 μm), and visual acuity of 20/32 or better in both eyes. Category 2 patients have mild or borderline, age-related macular features (multiple small drusen, single or nonextensive intermediate drusen (63-124 μm), pigment abnormalities, or any combination of these) in one or both eyes, and visual acuity of 20/32 or better in both eyes. Category 3 patients require the absence of advanced AMD in both eyes and at least one eye with visual acuity of 20/32 or better with at least one large drusen (125 μm), extensive (as measured by drusen area) intermediate drusen, or geographic atrophy (GA) that does not involve the center of the macula, or any combination of these. Category 4 patients have visual acuity of 20/32 or better and no advanced AMD in one eye, with the fellow eye having either lesions of advanced AMD, or visual acuity less than 20/32 with AMD abnormalities sufficient to explain reduced visual acuity as determined by examination of photographs. "Advanced AMD" is defined as having GA involving the center of the macula or features of choroidal neovascularization.

Multiple prospective cohort studies including the Beaver Dam Eye Study, the Blue Mountains Eye Study, and the Carotenoids and Age-related Eye Disease Study (CAREDS), have found diets higher in zinc, vitamin C, vitamin E and carotenoids are associated with a lower risk of AMD progression.[2-7] These observational studies, although limited by unmeasured confounding and potential recall bias, provided the rationale for controlled trials evaluating the efficacy of nutritional supplements in reducing the progression of AMD.

Our report focuses on the evidence documenting the potential benefits and harms of certain dietary supplements in patients with AMD. Recommendations to the Department of Veterans Affairs with regard to these supplements will have important implications to that patient population as well as to older U.S. adults. We conducted a systematic review of published literature to address the following key questions:

1) In patients with age-related macular degeneration, do nutritional supplements containing carotenoids, antioxidants, or omega-3 fatty acids alone or in combination prevent functional visual loss?

2) In adult populations, what are the harms of carotenoid, antioxidant, and omega-3 fatty acid supplementation?

METHODS

TOPIC DEVELOPMENT

The review was commissioned by the Department of Veterans Affairs' Evidence-based Synthesis Program. We conferred with VA and non-VA experts to select the patients and subgroups, interventions, outcomes, and setting addressed in the review. We addressed the following key questions in our review of the literature:

1) In patients with age-related macular degeneration, do nutritional supplements containing carotenoids, antioxidants, or omega-3 fatty acids alone or in combination prevent functional visual loss?

2) In adult populations, what are the harms of carotenoid, antioxidant, and omega-3 fatty acid supplementation?

The criteria for patient population, treatment and comparator interventions, outcomes of interest, and patient care setting are outlined below:

Patients: Adults with nonexudative age-related macular degeneration

Interventions: Carotenoids – zeaxanthin, lutein, beta-carotene
Antioxidants – zinc, vitamin E, vitamin C
Omega-3 fatty acids – alpha linolenic acid (C18:3n-3), docosahexaenoic acid
(DHA; C22:6n-3), eicosapentaenoic acid (EPA; C20:5n-3)

Comparators: Placebo

Outcomes: Vision loss, defined as visual impairment in the best eye as follows:
$\leq 20/60$ by Snellen acuity; or $\leq 6/18$ metric acuity; or doubling of the visual angle
(e.g. 20/50 to 20/100); or $\geq$ three lines of loss; or ≥ 15 letters lost (ETDRS chart); or,
progression to advanced disease (either central geographic atrophy or wet macular
degeneration). Note: A 3-line change in visual acuity (i.e. +/-15 letters) using the ETDRS
chart is equivalent to a doubling of the visual angle.
Other outcomes: quality of life and functional status

Setting: Outpatient

Figure 1 illustrates the analytic framework that guided our review and synthesis.

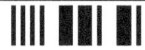

Nutritional Supplements for Age-related Macular Degeneration:
A Systematic Review   Evidence-based Synthesis Program

Figure 1. Analytic Framework

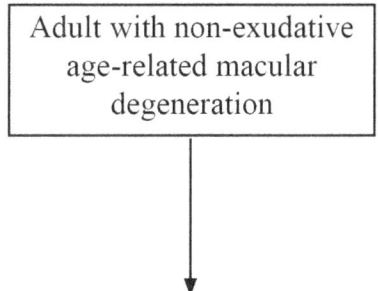

Adult with non-exudative
age-related macular
degeneration

Treatment interventions:
A. Carotenoids: zeaxanthin, lutein, beta-carotene
B. Antioxidants: zinc, vitamin E, vitamin C
C. Omega-3 fatty acids: alpha linolenic acid (C18:3n-3),
    docosahexaenoic acid (DHA; C22:6n-3),
    eicosapentaenoic acid (EPA; C20:5n-3)

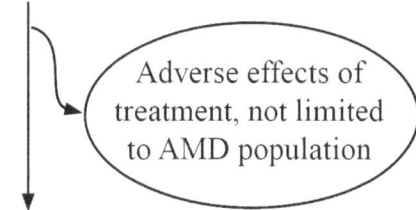

Adverse effects of
treatment, not limited
to AMD population

Outcomes:
- Vision loss: visual impairment in
  the best eye of >=20/60 Snellen;
  or >=3 lines or 15 letters loss; or
  progression to advanced AMD
- Quality of life
- Functional status

SEARCH STRATEGY

We conducted a search in Medline® Embase, Scopus, Conference Papers Index, and the
Cochrane Library (Cochrane Database of Systematic Reviews; Database of Abstracts of Reviews
of Effects; Cochrane Central Register of Controlled Trials) from 1947 or database inception
through February 2011. Appendix A provides the search strategy in detail. We obtained additional
articles from systematic reviews, reference lists of pertinent studies, reviews, editorials, and by
consulting experts. All citations were imported into an electronic database (EndNote X1).

STUDY SELECTION

Four reviewers assessed for relevance the abstracts of citations identified from literature
searches. Full-text articles of potentially relevant abstracts were retrieved for further review.
Each article retrieved was independently reviewed by two authors using the eligibility criteria
shown in Appendix B.

Eligible articles had English-language abstracts and provided primary data relevant to the key questions. Eligibility criteria varied depending on the question of interest, as described below.

To evaluate the efficacy of oral supplements, we considered prospective, controlled clinical trials comparing the effects of carotenoids, antioxidants, or omega-3 fatty acids (alone or in combination) with usual care or placebo on clinically significant vision loss, quality of life, or functional status among adults with age-related macular degeneration. We defined clinically important vision loss as any one of the following based on input from our Technical Expert Panel: ≤20/60 by Snellen acuity; or ≤6/18 metric acuity; or doubling of the visual angle (e.g. 20/50 to 20/100); or ≥ three lines of loss; or ≥15 letters lost; or progression to advanced disease (either central geographic atrophy or wet macular degeneration). We did not limit RCTs by sample size or duration of treatment.

We used a similar approach to evaluate the adverse effects of these oral supplements, but we also included studies of adults without AMD because the potential harms of oral supplements are not specific to those with AMD. Since nutritional supplements for AMD are intended for use over long periods of time and because clinically important harms not detected by AMD studies are unlikely to be evident in very small studies, we included only those studies with at least 24 weeks of follow-up and a sample size of 100 or more subjects (Appendix B).

DATA ABSTRACTION

From each study, we abstracted the following: study setting; number of subjects; population characteristics (including sex, age, race/ethnicity); treatment type, dosage and duration; type of control used; visual outcome results; proportion of subjects who progressed to severe AMD; quality of life and functional outcome results; adverse effects or treatments; and funding source.

STUDY QUALITY

Two reviewers independently assessed the quality of each AMD trial using a tool developed by the Cochrane Collaboration (Appendix C).[8] This tool asks the following questions about the methodologic characteristics of each study to guide assessment of the risk of bias:

- Was the allocation sequence adequately generated?
- Was allocation adequately concealed?
- Blinding of participants, personnel and outcome assessors: Was knowledge of the allocated intervention adequately prevented during the study?
- Were incomplete outcome data adequately addressed?
- Are reports of the study free of suggestion of selective outcome reporting?
- Was the study apparently free of other problems that could put it at a high risk of bias? (We assessed whether or not there were extreme baseline differences between groups.)

Disagreements were resolved through discussion. Each study was then given an overall summary assessment of low, high, or unclear risk of bias. The risk of bias within a given study can vary according to outcome. For instance, the risk of bias associated with lack of blinding might be low for mortality outcomes, but high for more subjective outcomes such as quality of life or symptom scores.

RATING THE BODY OF EVIDENCE

We assessed the overall body of evidence for each outcome by considering the consistency, coherence, and applicability across studies, as well as the internal validity of individual studies, using a method developed by the Grades of Recommendation, Assessment, Development, and Evaluation (GRADE) Working Group.[9]

DATA SYNTHESIS

We critically analyzed the strength of the evidence regarding both efficacy and adverse treatment effects, and compiled a qualitative synthesis of findings. We could not conduct a quantitative synthesis because the outcome measures, treatments, and populations differed substantially across trials.

PEER REVIEW

A draft version of this report was sent to the Technical Expert Panel and additional peer reviewers. We revised the report based on peer review feedback (Appendix D).

RESULTS

LITERATURE FLOW

We reviewed 4,335 titles and abstracts from the electronic search, and identified 22 additional references through manual searching of reference lists or from input from technical advisors.

After applying inclusion/exclusion criteria at the abstract level, 347 full-text articles were reviewed, as shown in Figure 2. Of the full-text articles, we rejected 308 that did not meet our inclusion criteria.

Figure 2. Literature Flow

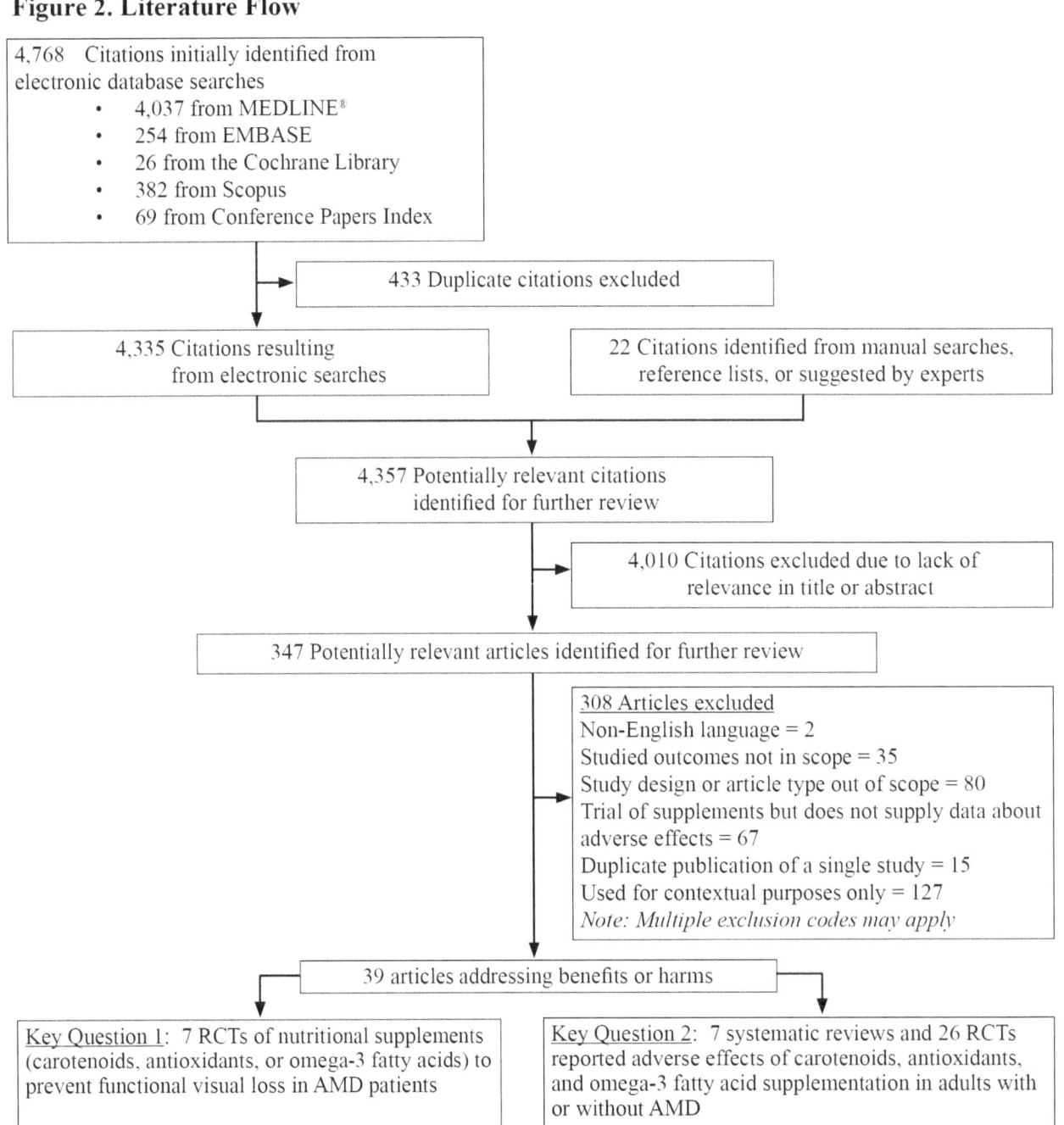

Nutritional Supplements for Age-related Macular Degeneration:
A Systematic Review   Evidence-based Synthesis Program

KEY QUESTION #1. In patients with age-related macular degeneration, do nutritional supplements containing carotenoids, antioxidants, or omega-3 fatty acids alone or in combination prevent functional visual loss?

Summary of findings

We identified seven randomized controlled trials (RCTs) of nutritional supplements in AMD patients. A significant effect in preventing functional loss was found only in the two largest trials.[10, 11] The weight of evidence was dominated by the Age Related Eye Disease Study (AREDS)[10] in terms of sample size (N=3640) and duration of follow-up (seven years). The sample sizes in the other six studies ranged from 60 to 164 subjects, with follow-up ranging from 6 to 24 months. Given that progression of AMD occurs slowly and with low frequency, the smaller studies might have been of insufficient duration or power to detect a treatment effect.

In the AREDS study, a beneficial effect was only observed among subjects with Categories 3 and 4 AMD, while no significant change was reported in mild AMD subjects (Category 1 or 2) in any of the three treatment arms compared with placebo. The protective effect of greatest magnitude among all of the supplement treatment arms was noted in the zinc plus antioxidant group OR=0.63 (99% CI; 0.44-0.92).

Detailed findings

Table 1 shows the detailed characteristics and findings of included studies.

Carotenoids

One randomized trial reported the effects of a supplemental carotenoid, lutein (10 mg/d), among subjects with AMD.[12] Subjects were randomized to lutein alone (N=29), lutein + antioxidants (OcuPower®; N=30) or placebo (N=31) for 12 months. The authors report very small increases in visual acuity in the lutein and lutein + antioxidants groups, but these changes were not clinically significant (<15 letters) after a one-year follow-up.

Antioxidants

Six RCTs evaluated the effects of antioxidant supplements in patients with Categories 2 to 4 AMD.[10-15] Three of these examined a mixture of antioxidant nutrients, including vitamin C, vitamin E, and some carotenoids such as beta carotene or quercetin. The remaining three studies used zinc alone in the form of zinc sulfate (200 mg/d),[11, 13] or as zinc monocysteine (50 mg/d).[14]

By far, the largest study was the multicenter AREDS trial which randomized 3,640 patients with Categories 2, 3 and 4 AMD into four treatment groups: antioxidants with carotenoids, zinc alone, antioxidants with carotenoids + zinc, or placebo.[10] The primary outcome was progression to advanced AMD (central geographic atrophy or choroidal neovascularization) and at least moderate functional visual loss, defined as the loss of ≥15 letters on the ETDRS logMAR chart. A secondary visual outcome was a decrease in the best corrected visual acuity score from baseline of 30 or more letters in a study eye (six lines or a quadrupling of the initial visual angle) and progression of disease to a visual acuity score worse than 20/100 in one or both eyes. Overall, in analyses limited to only those with Category 3 or 4 AMD, a reduction in functional visual loss was noted with either supplement alone or in combination.[10] Specifically, after five years of follow-up, the zinc/antioxidant combination significantly decreased the degree of functional vision loss (OR 0.63; 99% CI 0.44-0.92). A similar but smaller effect was noted with either supplement alone (zinc alone OR 0.75; 99% CI 0.53-1.07; antioxidants alone OR 0.79; 99% CI 0.55-1.13). On the other hand, antioxidants were not associated with benefit in the large subgroup of patients with Category 2 AMD (N = 1063) over seven years of follow-up. Of note, there was a very low rate of progression from Category 2 AMD to more advanced disease. Of patients with Category 2 AMD at baseline, 13 progressed to advanced AMD and 316 progressed to Category 3 or 4 AMD during the study. No significant differences in demographics, socioeconomic status, smoking status, or comorbidities were noted between the Category 2, 3 or 4 participants.

One additional trial found benefit from supplement use.[11] In this small trial, 174 patients with Category 3 or 4 AMD were randomized to either zinc sulfate supplements (200 mg/day) or placebo. Seventy-one subjects in the placebo and 80 subjects in the zinc group completed the two-year follow-up. Most patients had Category 3 or 4 AMD at baseline, and half the participants had baseline evidence of geographic atrophy. The placebo group was twice as likely as the zinc-supplemented group to demonstrate clinically significant vision loss (15.5% vs. 7.5%).

The other four studies were small (N = 56 or less), of relatively short duration (6 to 24 months), and did not report a clinically significant reduction in visual loss from supplement use.[12-15] Two of these trials were conducted in VA settings. One of the VA trials found the combination of lutein + antioxidants improved visual acuity, but not to a clinically significant degree.[12] Another small, multicenter VA trial evaluated the effects of a tablet containing a number of antioxidants and, similarly, found non-clinically significant improvement in visual acuity.[15] One small, non-VA trial of zinc supplementation found intervention patients had better visual acuity compared to the placebo group, but the difference was <15 letters on the ETDRS chart.[14] One other small single center trial found no difference in visual acuity between zinc supplement and placebo groups.[13]

Omega-3 fatty acids

One study examined the effects of supplemental omega-3 fatty acids, L-carnitine and coenzyme Q10 among subjects with AMD.[16] Most (93.6%) subjects in this study had "early" AMD at baseline; only 6.4 percent had Category 3 or 4 AMD. The study randomized subjects to omega-3 fatty acid supplement (N=52), or placebo (N=55). The change in visual acuity was measured after 12 months of supplementation. The report noted that omega-3 fatty acids slowed visual acuity loss, but not to a clinically significant degree (0.5 line change in Snellen acuity).

tional Supplements for Age-related Macular Degeneration: A Systematic Review

1. Characteristics and findings of controlled trials of nutritional supplements for age-related macular degeneration

r, year; setting	% male; race/ethnicity; mean age; smoking; comorbidities	Baseline visual acuity; % of population with Category 3 or 4 AMD at baseline	Treatment arms (daily dosage unless otherwise specified); N of subjects; duration of treatment	Visual acuity outcomes	Progression to severe AMD, % of subjects	Assessed risk of bias
enoids						
, 2004[12] North o and	96% male, white Mean age 74.4 Smoking: Lutein alone: 5.2 pack yrs +/-14.1; Placebo arm: 9.2 pack yrs +/-22.5 Comorbidities NR	Mean logMAR by treatment group: Lutein alone: R0.359 L0.279 Placebo: R0.445 L0.286	Lutein alone (10 mg non-esterified), N=29 Lutein plus antioxidants (OcuPower®), N=30 Placebo, N=31 12 months	Lutein alone: +5.4 Snellen (95% CI 2.7-9.0) p-value=0.01/ Placebo: -2.1 Snellen (95% CI -6.7-2.4) p-value not reported Effect size < 15 letters (i.e. not statistically nor clinically significant, p-values not reported)	NR	Low
idants alone or in combination with carotenoids, or other supplements						
S, nal ty US	44% male 96% white Mean age 69 yrs 8% current smokers 47% former smokers 9% baseline angina 6% taking DM meds 9% on lipid lowering meds 33% on HTN meds 11% dx with angina 8% prior CA dx	All eligible pts had signif AMD in one eye but the best eye had at least 20/32 vision; visual acuity was assessed by ETDRS chart. Younger pts 55-59 yrs were eligible only if they had Cat 3 or 4 AMD. Ocular media had to be clear and no other lesions as confounders present. 29% of subjects had Cat 2 40.2% had Cat 3 22.4% had Cat 4	Antioxidants alone (vit C, 500mg; vit E, 400 IU; beta carotene, 15mg), N=945 Antioxidants plus zinc, N=888 Placebo, N=903 8 years	(Reported only for Cat 3 & 4 at 5 years) Note: This data is reported as probability (or absolute event rate) of visual loss at 5 years; p-values are presented here for equivalent odds ratios reported in Table 5 of this AREDS report. **Visual loss** from 20/32 to <20/50 vision per ETDRS (a decrease in BVA from baseline of >=15 letters): Antioxidants alone: 26% p-value=0.07 Antioxidants plus zinc: 23% p-value=0.008 Placebo: 29% p-value not reported **Marked Visual Loss** from 20/32 to 20/100 in one eye (p-values not reported; rather odds ratios with 99% CI were reported): Antioxidants alone: 14% (OR, 0.80; 99% CI, 0.55-1.16) Antioxidants plus zinc: 12% (OR, 0.68; 99% CI, 0.46-1.01) Placebo: 17% (p-values not reported)	Subjects with Cat 3 & 4 who develop advanced AMD at 5 years: Antioxidants alone: 23% Antioxidants plus zinc: 20% Placebo: 28% Outcomes in Cat 2 subjects, treatment group NR: 15/1063 (1.4%) progressed to advanced AMD over 5 years; 316 (29.7%) advanced to Cat 3 or 4; no effect of treatment observed	Low
1996[15] edical	93% male Mean age 72 Smoking: placebo 0.1 pack/day; Ocuguard 0.06 pack/day 52% HTN; 31% CVD; 17% type 2 DM	Placebo: R eye logMAR 0.24 +/-0.03; L eye 0.24 +/- 0.03; Ocuguard: R eye 0.27 +/- 0.04; L eye 0.19 +/- 0.03	Ocuguard (20000 IU beta-carotene; 200 IU vit E; 750 mg vit C; 50 mg quercetin; 12.5 zinc; 50 ug selenium; 100 mg taurine; 25 mg vit B12; 100 ug chromium), N=39 Placebo, N=32	Placebo: -4 Snellen R eye; -15 Snellen L eye Antioxidant: -5 Snellen R eye; no change L eye Effect size <3 lines p-values not reported	NR	Low

r, year, setting	% male/ ethnicity; mean age; smoking; comorbidities	Baseline visual acuity; % of population with Category 3 or 4 AMD at baseline	Treatment arms (daily dosage unless otherwise specified); N of subjects; duration of treatment	Visual acuity outcomes	Progression to severe AMD, % of subjects	Assessed risk of bias
2004[12] cher, nder noids	See Richer, 2004 under Carotenoids	Mean logMAR by treatment group: Lutein plus antioxidants: R0.324 L0.303 Placebo: R0.445 L0.286	Lutein (10 mg non-esterified) plus antioxidants (2500 IU vit A; 15,000 IU vit C; 400 beta carotene; 1500 mg vit C; 400 IU vit D; 500 IU vit E; 50 mg vit B1; 10 mg vit B2; 70 mg vit B3; 50 mg vit B5; 50 mg vit B6; 500 ug B12; 800 ug folic acid 200 ug biotin; 500 mg ca++; 300 mg Mg; 75 ug Iodine; 25 mg zinc; 1 mg Cu; 2 mg Mn; 200 ug Se; 200 ug Cr; 75 ug Mb; 600 mg lycopene; 150 mg lipoic acid), N=30 Placebo, N=31 12 months	Lutein plus antioxidants: +3.5 Snellen (95% CI 0.8-6.1) Placebo: -2.1 Snellen (95% CI -6.7-2.4) effect size < 3 lines p-values not reported	NR	Low
one S, REDS, under dants	See AREDS, 2001 under Antioxidants	See AREDS, 2001 under Antioxidants	Zinc alone (80 mg as zinc oxide and 2 mg copper as cupric oxide), N= 904 Placebo, N=903 8 years	(Reported only for Cat 3 & 4 at 5 years) Note: This data is reported as probability (or absolute event rate) of visual loss at 5 years; p-values are presented here for equivalent odds ratios reported in Table 5 of this AREDS report. **Visual loss** from 20/32 to <20/50 vision per ETDRS (a decrease in BVA from baseline of >=15 letters): Zinc alone: 25% p-value=0.04 Placebo: 29% p-value not reported **Marked Visual Loss** from 20/32 to 20/100 in one eye(p-values not reported; rather odds ratios with 99% CI were reported): Zinc alone: 13% (OR, 0.75; 99% CI, 0.52-1.08), Placebo: 17% (p-values not reported)	Progression from baseline Cat 3 & 4 at 5 years: Zinc: 22% Placebo: 28%	Low
ome, center,	43% male Mean age 68 Ethnicity NR Smoking similar btw groups, NOS Zinc gp: 36% male 22.5% CVD, 33% HTN, 11% both CVD + HTN	Zinc group: VA >20/25 in 25/80 Placebo: VA >20/25 in 23/84	Zinc sulfate (200 mg/day; 100 mg bid) N=90 Placebo, N=84 24 months	Zinc vs placebo, Gain of 10 letters: 3/80 v 1/71 Loss of 10-14 letters 5/80 v 13/71 Loss of 15-19 letters 4/80 v 6/71 Loss of >20 letters 2/80 v 5/71 (p-values not reported)	NR	Low

16

tional Supplements for Age-related Macular Degeneration: A Systematic Review

or, year; setting	% male; race/ethnicity; mean age; smoking; comorbidities	Baseline visual acuity; % of population with Category 3 or 4 AMD at baseline	Treatment arms (daily dosage unless otherwise specified); N of subjects; duration of treatment	Visual acuity outcomes	Progression to severe AMD, % of subjects	Assessed risk of bias
ome, center, Orleans,	20% male 81% white 19% African American Mean age 73 Smoking NR Comorbidities NR	Placebo visual acuity (ETDRS logMAR) R eye: 40.297 +/-0.649 L eye: 39.270 +/-0.516 Treatment group visual acuity: R eye: 39.027 +/-0.672 L eye: 39.257 +/-0.585	Zinc monocysteine (50 mg/day; 25 mg bid), N=37 Placebo (bid), N=37 6 months	Zinc: 20/50 at baseline improved to 20/46 right eye and 20/47 left eye at 6 months (p-value=0.0001) Placebo group baseline vision 20/50 with no change over 6 months (p-value=0.0001)	NR	Low
996[13] center, a, a	42.9% male 100% white Mean age 72.3 +/-8 yrs 20% smoke 10 cigarettes/d 38% HTN	LogMAR(mean +-SD) Zinc: 0.073 +/-0.12 Placebo: 0.076 +/-0.13 72% high risk AMD 22% low risk AMD*	Zinc sulfate (200 mg), N=56 Placebo, N=56 24 months	LogMAR at 24 months trt N=37 0.046 +/-0.12 (p-value=0.52; placebo N=41 0.027 +/-0.14 effect size <15 letters (p-value not reported) Zinc: 20/22 at baseline to 20/22 at 24 months Placebo: 20/22 at baseline to 20/21 at 24 months	25% after 44.8 +-8.2 months	Low
a-3 fatty acids						
2005[16] center, ry	33% male Mean age 63 15.1% smokers Comorbidities NR	20/25-20/50 in worse eye: all had early AMD as part of inclusion criteria. 8/92 (8.7%) treatment grp and 4/96 (4.2%) of placebo had Cat 3 AMD at baseline (both eyes were considered for AMD progression, whereas only the worse eye was considered for visual acuity outcome)	Phototrop (proprietary compound of Acetyl-L-carnitine, ALC; n-3 FAs; and CoQ10), N=52 Placebo, N=55 12 months	Change in mean Snellen acuity, Phototrop vs placebo: Improved in 77% vs 55% (by .05 Snellen decimal) Deteriorated in 23% vs 45% (also by 0.05 Snellen decimal), p=0.015; OR 2.78 for deterioration, placebo vs active Tx.	Not reported...outcomes were measured as changes in drusen covered areas by photography	Low

iations: AMD = age-related macular degeneration; C = control; CA = cancer; ETDRS = Early Treatment Diabetic Retinopathy Study; logMAR= logarithm of the minimum angle of resolution, a ... for scoring visual acuity; Tx = Treatment; HTN = hypertension; N = number of subjects; NOS = not otherwise specified; NR = not reported.

-risk AMD" eyes were defined as eyes with a predominant drusen size of more than 125 /Ltm and/or a large drusen size of more than 250 /m and/or definite evidence of focal RPE ...eration and/or definite presence of drusen confluence. Eyes that did not exceed these limits were classified as "low-risk AMD" eyes.[13] Definitions of AREDS categories for AMD severity (AREDS No. 8):

ry 1: essentially free of age-related macular abnormalities, with a total drusen area less than 5 small drusen (<63 μm), and visual acuity of 20/32 or better in both eyes.

ry 2: mild or borderline age-related macular features (multiple small drusen, single or nonextensive intermediate drusen (63-124 μm), pigment abnormalities, or any combination of these) in 1 eyes, and visual acuity of 20/32 or better in both eyes.

ry 3: absence of advanced AMD in both eyes and at least 1 eye with visual acuity of 20/32 or better with at least 1 large drusen (125 μm), extensive (as measured by drusen area) intermediate or geographic atrophy (GA) that did not involve the center of the macula, or any combination of these.

ry 4: visual acuity of 20/32 or better and no advanced AMD (GA involving the center of the macula or features of choroidal neovascularization) in the study eye, and the fellow eye had either of advanced AMD or visual acuity less than 20/32 and AMD abnormalities sufficient to explain reduced visual acuity as determined by examination of photographs at the reading center.

Ongoing studies

The National Institute of Health (NIH) has commissioned the National Eye Institute to conduct the Age-Related Eye Disease Study 2 (AREDS II), and the trial is currently underway.[17] Enrollment of subjects began in September 2006 and is now complete. Approximately 4,200 subjects will be followed for five years with an estimated completion date of December 2012. Subjects between ages 50 and 85, with clear enough media for retinal photography (e.g. no significant cataracts), and who had various stages of macular degeneration are included. The study design is a double-blinded RCT of five-year duration, with the primary outcome measure of progression to advanced AMD in subjects at moderate to high risk for progression (e.g. Categories 3 and 4 AMD). Secondary outcome measures pertinent to our review are: progression to moderate vision loss; adverse events; and, effect of DHA/EPA on cardiovascular morbidity and mortality. The purpose of the study is to evaluate the effect of lutein and zeaxanthin (two dietary xanthophylls), and two omega-3 fatty acids DHA and EPA on these outcome measures. Additionally, the treatment arms will evaluate the effects of eliminating beta-carotene from the original AREDS formulation of antioxidants (500 mg vitamin C; 400 IU vitamin E; and 15 mg beta carotene), and/or lowering the zinc component of the supplement (previously 80 mg zinc as zinc oxide, and 2 mg copper as cupric oxide). All participants are offered additional treatment with the original AREDS formulation (now considered the standard of care). It is doubtful whether this study will be able to address the more subtle loss of functional vision in lower risk patients upon which our review was focused. This is the result of the natural history of early AMD, which is characterized by long duration and slow progression of the disease. The sample size of the AREDS II will again cause this study to statistically dominate similar studies of these outcome measures for the foreseeable future.

KEY QUESTION #2. In adult populations, what are the harms of carotenoid, antioxidant, and omega-3 fatty acid supplementation?

Seven systematic reviews examined the adverse effects of oral supplements in 56 RCTs. One review included trials of adults with AMD,[18] while other reviews included a range of study populations. One review examined mortality in trials of vitamin E.[19] Two reviews examined the risk of lung cancer in trials of beta-carotene,[20, 21] and one of these reviews also examined prospective observational studies of carotenoids for lung cancer incidence.[20] Three reviews included studies of various supplements (B-carotene, vitamin A, vitamin C, vitamin E, alpha-tocopherol, zinc), alone or in combination, to examine the effects on colorectal adenoma,[22] gastrointestinal cancers,[23] and prostate cancer.[24]

Thirty-three large (N >1000) RCTs with more than one year of follow-up were accounted for by the prior systematic reviews. Because of their size and length of follow-up, these trials provide the richest source of information about potential harms of these supplements. As their results are well represented in prior reviews, we focus below on the findings of previous evidence syntheses, supplemented with data from our own review of primary studies of this added new information. In addition to existing systematic reviews, we examined 173 publications from 41 trials for reports of adverse effects of oral supplements in adults, not limited to patients with AMD.

Summary of findings

Vitamin E at high doses (>=400 IU/day) may be associated with increased risk of mortality, congestive heart failure, and prostate cancer.

Beta-carotene may be associated with an increased risk of lung cancer among active smokers. In the Beta-Carotene and Retinol Efficacy Trial (CARET) and Alpha-Tocopherol and Beta-Carotene (ATBC) trials, beta-carotene was associated with increased mortality and increased risk of lung cancer among smokers. Two other large trials, the Women's Health Study (WHS) and the Physicians' Health Study (PHS), did not find an excess risk of lung cancer among smokers using beta-carotene, but a meta-analysis combining these four studies determined that the overall risk of lung cancer among current smokers treated with beta-carotene was significantly elevated (OR 1.24 (95% CI, 1.10-1.39)). No increase in lung cancer incidence was observed among former smokers and nonsmokers in these studies. In prospective cohort studies that used lower doses than RCTs, a small inverse association between carotenoids and lung cancer among current smokers has been observed.

Zinc was associated with urinary tract infections and hospital admissions due to genitourinary causes in one study.

Yellowish discoloration of the skin was frequently reported in trials of beta-carotene, and has also been noted in trials of lutein. Gastrointestinal symptoms were also commonly reported in trials of various supplements.

Detailed findings

Mortality

A systematic review of various supplements (beta-carotene, vitamin A, vitamin C, vitamin E, and selenium in combination) found that the relative risk (RR) of all-cause mortality was significantly increased with antioxidants compared with placebo (RR 1.05, 95% CI 1.02-1.07), in a meta-analysis that combined 13 trials with low risk of bias.[23] There was significant heterogeneity among the trials, however, and the combined estimate appeared to be driven by two large studies of beta-carotene that contributed 52 percent of the weight in the analysis: the ATBC study,[25] which included 29,133 male smokers; and the CARET study,[26] which enrolled 18,314 smokers, former smokers, and workers exposed to asbestos.

In ATBC, there were marginally significant increases in mortality after 6.1 mean years of treatment in the group that received 20 mg/day beta-carotene alone (RR 1.08 (95% CI 0.99-1.19)) and the group that received 20 mg/day beta-carotene plus a low dose (50 IU/day) of vitamin E (RR 1.10 (95% CI 1.00-1.21)), whereas mortality was not elevated in the group that received vitamin E alone (RR 1.02, 95% CI 0.93-1.12).[25] In the CARET study, the active treatment group combined 30 mg beta-carotene together with 25,000 IU vitamin A and was associated with a 17 percent increase in mortality compared with placebo after four years of treatment (RR 1.17, 95% CI 1.03-1.33).[26] A post-intervention analysis of the CARET study determined that the increase in all-cause mortality in the beta-carotene/vitamin A group remained elevated six years after the trial had ended, although the magnitude of risk had diminished and become less significant (RR 1.08, 95% CI 0.99-1.17).[26]

A systematic review of vitamin E included 19 trials stratified by dosage (<400 IU/day or >=400 IU/day).[19] Low-dose vitamin E (16.5 to 330 IU/day) had no significant effect on all-cause mortality in a meta-analysis of eight trials. High-dose vitamin E (400 to 2000 IU/day) was associated with a significant increase in all-cause mortality in a meta-analysis of 11 trials. The risk ratio was 1.04 (95% CI 1.01-1.07, p=0.035) and the pooled risk increase was 39 deaths per 10,000 persons (95% CI 3-74 per 10,000, p=0.035) compared with controls. The reviewers conducted a dose-response analysis that showed a statistically significant trend of increased mortality with vitamin E dosage >150 IU/day.[19]

Cancer

Lung cancer

A systematic review of four RCTs examined the effects of beta-carotene (20 to 30 mg/day) on lung cancer incidence, stratified by smoking status.[21] Among current smokers, lung cancer incidence was significantly increased with beta-carotene supplementation in the ATBC[27] and CARET[28] studies, but not significantly increased in the PHS[29] and WHS[30] studies. Although the WHS study was terminated early after a median beta-carotene exposure of 2.1 years, (compared with 4 years in CARET, 6.1 years in ATBC, and 12 years in PHS) a meta-analysis combining the four studies determined that the overall risk of lung cancer among current smokers treated with beta-carotene was significantly increased (OR 1.24 (95% CI 1.10-1.39)).[21] Three of the studies (CARET, PHS, and WHS) included former smokers, and in this subgroup there was no association between beta-carotene and lung cancer incidence in any of the three studies (pooled OR 1.10, 95% CI 0.84-1.45).[21] Former smokers were defined in the CARET study as individuals who smoked within the past 15 years but quit smoking more than six years prior to the study[28], whereas individuals were classified as former smokers in PHS and WHS if they had smoked in the past but had quit at the onset of the study. No significant increase in lung cancer incidence was observed among nonsmokers (OR 0.73, 95% CI 0.33-1.59).[21]

Another review of carotenoids and lung cancer incidence examined data from six RCTs and 24 prospective observational studies.[20] The review noted the increased risk of lung cancer among smokers in the CARET and ATBC studies, but found a small inverse association between carotenoids and lung cancer among current smokers in prospective cohort studies. The reviewers noted that the RCTs used beta-carotene at doses 5 to 10 times greater than normal dietary intake, and suggested that beta-carotene may accelerate the growth of already initiated cells if administered in later stages of the carcinogenic process.[20]

A follow-up analysis of the ATBC study containing updated cancer data determined that the excess risk of lung cancer associated with beta-carotene during the trial period was attenuated (RR 1.16, 95% CI 0.97-1.40)[25] compared with the initial findings (RR 1.19, 95% CI 1.04-1.36)[27] that were used in the meta-analysis cited above.[21] The follow-up of the ATBC study examined post-intervention cancer incidence and determined that the excess risk of lung cancer among beta-carotene recipients was no longer evident four to six years after ending the intervention (RR 1.06, 95% CI 0.94-1.20).[25]

Prostate cancer

A systematic review and meta-analysis examined the incidence of prostate cancer with vitamin E in five large RCTs (N of subjects ranging from 9,541 to 35,533) with treatment duration of four

Nutritional Supplements for Age-related Macular Degeneration:
A Systematic Review   Evidence-based Synthesis Program

to eight years.[24] The pooled analysis showed no significant findings (HR 0.96, 95% CI 0.85-1.08) although the dosage and effects of vitamin E varied among the trials. The ATBC trial used a low dose of vitamin E (50 IU daily) and found a significantly protective effect against prostate cancer,[27] while the Selenium and Vitamin E Cancer Prevention Trial (SELECT) administered 400 IU/day and found a marginally elevated risk.[31]. The other three trials of vitamin E included in the meta-analysis administered 400 IU daily or every other day, and found neutral effects on prostate cancer incidence.

Data from follow-up studies of the ATBC and SELECT trials showed an upward shift in the risk of prostate cancer associated with vitamin E. The initial analysis of the SELECT trial based on 235,689 person-years of follow-up reported a 13 percent increased risk of prostate cancer with vitamin E (HR 1.13, 99% CI 0.95-1.35).[31] A post-trial analysis, which included an additional 54,464 person-years since the primary report, determined that the overall risk of prostate cancer among men in the Vitamin E group had increased to 17 percent above placebo (HR 1.17, 99% CI 1.004-1.36, p=0.008).[32] The study investigators determined that the absolute increase in risk of prostate cancer per 1000 person-years was 1.6 for subjects treated with vitamin E. The significantly protective effect of vitamin E on prostate cancer (RR 0.66, 95% CI 0.52-0.86) initially observed in the ATBC study diminished to non-significance during the six-year post-trial observation period (RR 0.88, 95% CI 0.76-1.03).[25]

No significant effects on incidence or mortality from prostate cancer were found in two RCTs of vitamin C, and in three RCTs of beta-carotene.[24]

Gastrointestinal cancer
A systematic review that examined the effects of various supplements (beta-carotene, vitamin A, vitamin C, vitamin E, and selenium, alone or in combination) among 20 RCTs found no effect on incidence of gastrointestinal cancers among 12 good-quality trials.[23]

Colorectal adenoma
A systematic review of various supplements (beta-carotene, vitamin A, vitamin C, vitamin E, and selenium, alone or in combination) found mixed effects on the development of colorectal adenoma among eight RCTs. Stratifying the studies by methodological quality, the review determined that antioxidant supplements appeared to increase the risk of colorectal adenoma in three low-bias risk trials (RR 1.2, 95% CI 0.99-1.4) while an opposite, significantly protective effect was observed in five high-bias risk trials (0.59, 95% CI 0.47-0.74).[23]

Cardiovascular disease

In the ATBC trial, low-dose vitamin E supplementation (50 IU/day alpha-tocopherol) decreased the risk of cerebral infarction but increased the risk of fatal hemorrhagic stroke among smokers. The study authors noted that the overall net effects of vitamin E on total stroke were nonsignificant.[33] A systematic review that included 10 trials of vitamin E (alone or combined with other supplements) concluded that vitamin E did not significantly affect the risk of hemorrhagic stroke (RR 1.01, 95% CI 0.82-1.23).[23]

In the GISSI-Prevenzione trial of post-infarction patients, vitamin E (300 mg/day for 3.5 years, open-label) increased the risk of the combined outcome of CHF hospitalization or death in patients with left ventricular dysfunction (HR 1.50, 95% CI 1.03-2.20) but not in those with preserved systolic function.[34]

In the HOPE trial, a double-blinded RCT of vitamin E (400 IU daily for a mean of 4.5 years) in 9,541 patients with DM, CVD, or renal insufficiency, CHF (i.e., hospitalization or death due to CHF, or use of an ACE inhibitor for the diagnosis of CHF) was increased with vitamin E supplementation (RR 1.13, 95% CI 1.01-1.26).[35] The increased CHF risk associated with vitamin E was found at extended follow-up (median 7 years; RR 1.19, 95% CI 1.05-1.35).[35]

An open-label trial of fish oil consumption in 3,114 men with angina observed a marginally significant increased risk of cardiac death at three to nine years among subjects advised to consume oily fish or fish oil capsules twice a week.[36] This study was methodologically limited by the lack of blinding, and the inability to determine the level of compliance with the dietary advice and other confounding factors.

In a double-blinded RCT of fish oil supplementation (6 g/day of n-3-fatty acids) for six months following coronary angioplasty in 205 patients, restenosis was non-significantly increased in the fish oil group (RR 1.7, 95% CI 0.9-3.4).[37] This effect was not observed in other studies of restenosis after coronary angioplasty[38, 39] or atrial fibrillation.[40]

Other adverse effects

Respiratory tract infections
In a double-blinded RCT of vitamin E (200 mg/dL/day for 15 months) among non-institutionalized individuals aged 60+, the incidence of respiratory tract infections did not differ with treatment. Among those who experienced a respiratory infection, however, individuals who received vitamin E had longer illness duration, more symptoms, and a higher frequency of fever and restriction of activity.[41] The authors of the study suggested that supplementation with vitamin E may improve immune response, and that the observed effect of vitamin E on illness severity might reflect a more active immune response.[41]

Urinary tract infections
Subjects treated with zinc (80 mg as zinc oxide and 2 mg copper as cupric oxide, daily, with 6.3 years mean follow-up) in the AREDS study experienced significantly more urinary tract infections compared with non-zinc treated subjects, particularly women (2.3% vs 0.4%, RR 5.77, 95% CI 1.30-25.66, p=0.013). There were more hospital admissions due to genitourinary causes, particularly among men (RR 1.26, 95% CI 1.07-1.50, p=0.008).[42]

Yellowish discoloration of the skin (carotenodermia)
Beta-carotene was significantly associated with yellowing of the skin in a systematic review that included five RCTs of beta-carotene,[24] as well as the AREDS study.[10] Another systematic review that included nine RCTs of beta-carotene determined that transient yellowing of the skin was increased but not to a statistically significant degree (RR 1.85, 95% CI 0.74-4.67).[23] In a trial of beta-carotene (15,000 IU), vitamin C (250 mg), and vitamin E (350 IU) taken together (2 capsules/2x daily) for six months following coronary angioplasty, yellow skin pigmentation was observed in 56 percent of patients taking multivitamins, but the significance of this finding relative to the placebo group in this study was not specified.[43]

Lutein has also been associated with carotenodermia. A narrative review of carotenoids[44] cited two trials of lutein in which this effect occurred, at daily doses of 15 mg for 4 to 5 months.[45, 46]

Gastrointestinal symptoms

A systematic review of 10 RCTs of antioxidant supplements to prevent or delay progression of AMD reported that gastrointestinal symptoms were the most common adverse effect that led to withdrawal from studies.[18] In a trial of beta-carotene (15,000 IU), vitamin C (250 mg), and vitamin E (350 IU) taken together (2 capsules/2x daily) for six months following coronary angioplasty, diarrhea occurred more frequently among the multivitamin group compared to placebo.[43] A systematic review of beta-carotene trials found increases in minor gastrointestinal (GI) symptoms.[24] A greater incidence of GI upset was also reported in at least two other trials: a trial of fatty acid supplementation (2 capsules/2x daily containing 280 mg of gamma-linolenic acid and 45 mg eicosapentaenoic acid) in patients with intermittent claudication,[47] and in a trial of beta-carotene (15,000 IU), vitamin C (250 mg), and vitamin E (350 IU) taken together (2 capsules/2x daily) for six months following coronary angioplasty.[43]

Anemia

More zinc-treated subjects self-reported the occurrence of anemia (13.2 vs 1.2%, p=0.004) in the AREDS study. This perceived effect was not supported by laboratory values, however, as serum hematocrit levels showed no significant differences between treatment groups.[10]

DISCUSSION

We conducted a systematic review of the benefits and harms of nutritional supplements for treatment of AMD. We found good evidence mainly from one large RCT that supplementation with carotenoids and antioxidants decreased the risk of functional vision loss among patients with Category 3 or 4 AMD. One smaller RCT also found zinc supplementation may decrease the risk of clinically significant visual loss among patients with Category 3 or 4 AMD, but six other RCTs found no clinically significant benefit from nutritional supplements in AMD patients. The effects of carotenoids or omega-3-fatty acids alone have not been well-studied.

It is likely that the discrepant findings reflect, at least in part, the size, length of follow-up, and patient characteristics in these six studies not finding benefit. These studies all included fewer than 200 patients each, were conducted over a relatively short time frame, and included large proportions of patients with mild AMD.

We also found evidence of significant potential harm from some nutritional supplements. Carotenoids such as beta-carotene have been associated with an estimated 24 percent increased risk of lung cancer among smokers. Similar to the studies of potential benefits, the evidence for harms is driven primarily by two large trials, ATBC and CARET. The release of the results regarding beta-carotene and lung cancer risk from ATBC in 1994[27] and CARET in 1996[28] caused an amendment to be made to the ongoing AREDS study, in which smokers were offered a chance to change their randomization of treatment supplements category to one which included either zinc alone or placebo. This concern also has been addressed in the subsequent AREDS II study, now underway, which is discussed below under Future Studies.[48]

Higher doses of vitamin E (>400 IU per day) have been associated with an estimated four percent increase in mortality; a 13 to 17 percent increase in risk of prostate cancer; and a 13 to 50 percent increase in risk of congestive heart failure among those with existing CVD risk factors such as left ventricular dysfunction, diabetes mellitus, recent myocardial infarction, or renal insufficiency.

Whether the balance of benefits and harms favors supplementation in AMD patients likely depends on the population being considered. There is strong evidence for benefit in patients with more advanced AMD; and in these patients, the very small risk of harm is likely to be outweighed by the potential benefit. Using the AREDS data, one can calculate the number needed to treat with supplements to prevent one patient from developing clinically significant visual loss, as 33 over five years. In a population of patients with comorbid cardiovascular disease, 256 would need to be treated with supplements (which include vitamin E) to cause one excess death.[19]

The role of nutritional supplementation in patients with mild AMD is unclear. The natural history of mild AMD is one of slow progression. Among 1,117 participants with Category 1 AMD at baseline in the AREDS study, only five (0.45%) participants developed advanced AMD during 6.3 mean years of follow-up. Among 1,063 subjects with Category 2 AMD at baseline, only 13 (1.2%) subjects had significant vision loss related to AMD, and 28 (2.6%) participants progressed to Category 3 or 4.[10] There was no detectable effect on vision loss in any of the treatment arms among these subjects, given the very slow rate of disease progression in mild AMD. It is unclear, however, whether the rate of progression from mild to advanced AMD increases with age. It

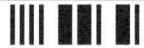

Nutritional Supplements for Age-related Macular Degeneration:
A Systematic Review   Evidence-based Synthesis Program

is possible that nutritional supplementation for mild AMD may yield more detectable benefit to those over age 85 compared with younger individuals. These aged individuals make up the fastest growing demographic in the United States. The natural progression of AMD in this age group warrants further study.

Since AMD patients are likely to be older and have additional medical comorbidities, many would be at risk for some of the potential harms associated with supplementation. Because of the very slow rate of disease progression in patients with mild AMD, the lack of evidence of benefit in these patients and the potential for harm – especially amongst those with baseline medical comorbidities – the current literature does not support widespread use of these supplements for mild AMD. The balance of benefits and harms in patients with Category 3 or 4 AMD and limited life expectancy is unclear. Because the benefits of nutritional supplements do take several years to accrue, it is unclear that their use in patients with limited life expectancy is indicated.

Our findings concur with and add to the findings of similar reviews. A recent Cochrane collaborative review found evidence for modest benefit of antioxidant, vitamin and mineral supplementation reducing the progression of AMD in people with moderate to severe signs of the disease, and no evidence that subjects with early signs of the disease show a treatment benefit.[18] Our findings add to prior reviews in that we looked at a broader group of studies to examine the potential harms of supplements because the potential risks are not limited to only those with AMD, making studies including all older adults relevant to the question of harms.

FUTURE STUDIES

Based on the progression observed in AREDS among subjects with Category 2 AMD, we estimate a study enrolling 17,000 subjects followed over five years would be needed to detect a clinically significant difference in visual loss between subjects treated with antioxidants + zinc versus a placebo. Such a study is unlikely to be funded and completed in the near future. The natural history of AMD is a very slow and lengthy progression from retinal evidence of disease to functional vision loss. Not all patients with evidence of retinal disease have vision impairment that interferes with functional status. In other words, subtle changes in retinal function due to AMD may cause visual disability that is not well reflected on the basis of visual acuity measurements alone. Well-validated intermediate markers of functional vision loss would be useful. Well-designed prospective cohort studies of patients with mild AMD could elucidate the types of intermediate findings that could accurately predict future clinically significant vision loss. In addition, studies would need to confirm that these findings are consistent when measured across large groups of patients.

Given the relative lack of information about the effects of xanthophylls, carotenoids, and omega-3 fatty acids, future trials should be considered to assess the effects of these supplements in AMD patients. The results of the ongoing AREDS II trial should help to address the current gaps in evidence about the effects of the xanthophyll and omega-3-fatty acids. In addition, the AREDS II trial interventions will include four variations of the original AREDS formula for randomization. However, smokers in the study will be randomized to only groups 2 or 3 since neither of these two groups' supplements includes beta-carotene. The only variation between these two groups is the high or low Zinc content. This comprises a "smokers" subset of AREDS II.[48]

Previous and current studies, including the ongoing AREDS II trial, have focused on functional vision loss and AMD progression as the principal outcomes of interest. The large majority of patients with AMD, however, may suffer from more subtle visual disabilities that may, nevertheless, profoundly alter their visual functioning, such as losing their ability to safely operate a motor vehicle. It is important to emphasize that these patients, while visually impaired, may still record less than clinically significant visual loss as measured by visual acuity. Evidence is lacking as to whether quality of life outcomes and activities of daily living benefit from treatment, and further study of these outcome measures is warranted.

CONCLUSIONS

Evidence of benefit from supplementation with carotenoids and antioxidants on functional vision loss in patients with AMD is based mainly on the results of one large trial. The observed benefit occurred only among subjects with Category 3 or 4 AMD. There is evidence for a low risk of harm from some nutritional supplements at high doses. As with any clinical intervention, the balance of benefits and harms regarding supplementation in AMD patients depends upon the population being considered. Given that AMD patients are older and have additional medical comorbidities, many would be at risk for some of the potential harms associated with supplementation. The precautionary principle should be observed while further evidence evolves. Table 2 summarizes the evidence regarding the benefits and harms of oral supplements for AMD.

While our report notes the uncertainty in the conclusions of many of the included studies, reasonable recommendations can be extended:

- Carotenoid and antioxidants supplements significantly decrease visual loss and can be recommended for patients with Categories 3 and 4 AMD.
- Current literature does not support the use of these supplements for patients with mild AMD.
- Certain nutritional supplements have significant potential harms:
    - Increased mortality and congestive heart failure in high risk patients with vitamin E.
    - Increased risk of prostate cancer with vitamin E.
    - Increased risk of lung cancer among smokers with beta-carotene.

Table 2. Summary of the evidence on the effects of nutritional supplements for age-related macular degeneration

Outcome	Treatment	Population	Effect*	GRADE Classification†	Comment
Functional vision loss	Carotenoids	Early AMD	(~)	Low	Single study (N=90) found a small increase in visual acuity after 12 months, but the improvement was not clinically significant (i.e. <15 letters).[12]
	Antioxidants‡	Categories 3-4 AMD	(+)	Moderate	Evidence of benefit from 1 large multicenter trial[10] and one smaller trial.[11] 4 small trials found neutral effects on functional vision loss.[12-15]
	Antioxidants	Category 2 AMD	(~)	Low	No evidence of benefit after 7 years of treatment in 1 large multicenter trial that included 1,063 Category 2 subjects.[10]
	Omega-3 fatty acids	Early AMD (94% in Categories 1- 2)	(~)	Very Low	One study found evidence of slowed visual acuity loss but not to a clinically significant degree. Very few subjects in this study (6.4%) had Categories 3-4 AMD.[16]
Quality of life	Carotenoids	AMD	(~)	Low	No significant findings on night driving in one study (N=90).[12]
	Antioxidants	N/A	(0)	N/A	No evidence.
	Omega-3 fatty acids	N/A	(0)	N/A	No evidence.
Mortality	Beta-carotene	Smokers	(–)	Moderate	High-dose beta-carotene (20 to 30 mg/day) was linked with increased mortality in 2 large trials in smokers and asbestos workers.[25, 26]
	Vitamin E	General population	(–)	High	High-dose vitamin E (>=400 IU/day) was associated with a slight increase in mortality in a meta-analysis of 11 trials.[19]
Lung cancer	Beta-carotene	Smokers	(–)	Moderate	High-dose beta-carotene (20 to 30 mg/day) was linked with increased lung cancer incidence among smokers in a meta-analysis of 4 large trials.[21] No increase in lung cancer was observed among former and non-smokers.
Prostate cancer	Vitamin E	General population	(–)	Low	High-dose vitamin E (400 IU/day) was associated with an increase in prostate cancer in one study.[31]
Gastro-intestinal cancers	Antioxidants	General population	(~)	High	Supplements had no effect on incidence of gastrointestinal cancers in a meta-analysis of 12 good-quality trials.[23]
Congestive heart failure	Vitamin E	DM, CVD, or post-infarction	(–)	Low	Vitamin E (300-400 IU/day) was linked with increased CHF hospitalization in 2 trials of high-risk patients.[34, 35]
Urinary tract infections (UTIs)	Zinc	AMD	(–)	Low	Zinc (80 mg/day) was associated with more UTIs and hospital admissions due to genitourinary causes compared with non-zinc treated subjects in one large study.[42]

Outcome	Treatment	Population	Effect*	GRADE Classification†	Comment
Yellowing of the skin	Beta-carotene Lutein	AMD and general population	(−)	High	Transient yellowing of the skin was frequently reported in trials of beta-carotene[24] and in two trials of lutein[44]
Gastro-intestinal (GI) symptoms	Antioxidants	AMD	(−)	High	GI symptoms were the most common adverse effect that led to withdrawal from studies, according to a systematic review of 10 RCTs of antioxidant supplements for AMD.[18]

GRADE = Grades of Recommendation, Assessment, Development, and Evaluation; ICU = intensive care unit; RCT = randomized controlled trial; AMD = age-related macular degeneration; CHF = congestive heart failure.

* Effect: (+) benefit; (−) harm; (~) mixed findings/no effect; (0) no evidence.

† GRADE classification: high = further research is very unlikely to change our confidence on the estimate of effect; moderate = further research is likely to have an important impact on our confidence in the estimate of effect and may change the estimate; low = further research is very likely to have an important impact on our confidence in the estimate of effect and is likely to change the estimate; very low = any estimate of effect is very uncertain.

‡ Trials of antioxidants included treatment with antioxidants alone or combined with carotenoids or other supplements.

REFERENCES

1.   Friedman DS, O'Colmain BJ, Munoz B, et al. Prevalence of age-related macular degeneration in the United States. *Archives of Ophthalmology.* Apr 2004;122(4):564-572.

2.   Augood C, Chakravarthy U, Young I, et al. Oily fish consumption, dietary docosahexaenoic acid and eicosapentaenoic acid intakes, and associations with neovascular age-related macular degeneration. *American Journal of Clinical Nutrition.* Aug 2008;88(2):398-406.

3.   Flood V, Smith W, Wang JJ, Manzi F, Webb K, Mitchell P. Dietary antioxidant intake and incidence of early age-related maculopathy: the Blue Mountains Eye Study. *Ophthalmology.* Dec 2002;109(12):2272-2278.

4.   Mares JA, Voland RP, Sondel SA, et al. Healthy lifestyles related to subsequent prevalence of age-related macular degeneration. *Archives of Ophthalmology.* Apr 2011;129(4):470-480.

5.   Mares-Perlman JA, Klein R, Klein BE, et al. Association of zinc and antioxidant nutrients with age-related maculopathy. *Archives of Ophthalmology.* Aug 1996;114(8):991-997.

6.   Moeller SM, Parekh N, Tinker L, et al. Associations between intermediate age-related macular degeneration and lutein and zeaxanthin in the Carotenoids in Age-related Eye Disease Study (CAREDS): ancillary study of the Women's Health Initiative. *Archives of Ophthalmology.* Aug 2006;124(8):1151-1162.

7.   VandenLangenberg GM, Mares-Perlman JA, Klein R, Klein BE, Brady WE, Palta M. Associations between antioxidant and zinc intake and the 5-year incidence of early age-related maculopathy in the Beaver Dam Eye Study. *American Journal of Epidemiology.* Jul 15 1998;148(2):204-214.

8.   Higgins JPT, Altman DG, editors. Chapter 8: Assessing risk of bias in included studies. In: Higgins JPT, Green S (editors). Cochrane Handbook for Systematic Reviews of Interventions. 2008;Version 5.0.1 [updated September 2008]. The Cochrane Collaboration, 2008. Available from www.cochrane-handbook.org.

9.   Guyatt G, Oxman AD, Akl EA, et al. GRADE guidelines: 1. Introduction-GRADE evidence profiles and summary of findings tables. *Journal of Clinical Epidemiology.* Apr 2011;64(4):383-394.

10.   Age-Related Eye Disease Study Research Group. A randomized, placebo-controlled, clinical trial of high-dose supplementation with vitamins C and E, beta carotene, and zinc for age-related macular degeneration and vision loss: AREDS report no. 8. *Archives of Ophthalmology.* Oct 2001;119(10):1417-1436.

11.   Newsome DA, Swartz M, Leone NC, Elston RC, Miller E. Oral zinc in macular degeneration. *Archives of Ophthalmology.* Feb 1988;106(2):192-198.

12.   Richer S, Stiles W, Statkute L, et al. Double-masked, placebo-controlled, randomized trial of lutein and antioxidant supplementation in the intervention of atrophic age-related macular degeneration: the Veterans LAST study (Lutein Antioxidant Supplementation Trial). *Optometry.* Apr 2004;75(4):216-230.

13.   Stur M, Tittl M, Reitner A, Meisinger V. Oral zinc and the second eye in age-related macular degeneration. *Investigative Ophthalmology & Visual Science.* Jun 1996;37(7):1225-1235.

14.   Newsome DA. A randomized, prospective, placebo-controlled clinical trial of a novel zinc-monocysteine compound in age-related macular degeneration. *Current Eye Research.* Jul 2008;33(7):591-598.

15.   Richer S. Multicenter ophthalmic and nutritional age-related macular degeneration study--part 2: antioxidant intervention and conclusions. *Journal of the American Optometric Association.* Jan 1996;67(1):30-49.

16.   Feher J, Kovacs B, Kovacs I, Schveoller M, Papale A, Balacco Gabrieli C. Improvement of visual functions and fundus alterations in early age-related macular degeneration treated with a combination of acetyl-L-carnitine, n-3 fatty acids, and coenzyme Q10. *Ophthalmologica.* May-Jun 2005;219(3):154-166.

17.   Age-Related Eye Disease Study 2 Investigators. Age-Related Eye Disease Study 2 (AREDS2): A Multi-Center, Randomized Trial of Lutein, Zeaxanthin and Omega-3 Long-Chain Polyunsaturated Fatty Acids (Docosahexaenoic Acid [DHA] and Eicosapentaenoic Acid [EPA]) in Age-Related Macular Degeneration *ClinicalTrials.gov identifier: NCT00345176 (Ongoing study).*

18.   Evans J. Antioxidant supplements to prevent or slow down the progression of AMD: a systematic review and meta-analysis. *Eye.* Jun 2008;22(6):751-760.

19.   Miller ER, 3rd, Pastor-Barriuso R, Dalal D, et al. Meta-analysis: high-dosage vitamin E supplementation may increase all-cause mortality. *Annals of Internal Medicine.* Jan 4 2005;142(1):37-46.

20.   Gallicchio L, Boyd K, Matanoski G, et al. Carotenoids and the risk of developing lung cancer: a systematic review. *American Journal of Clinical Nutrition.* Aug 2008;88(2):372-383.

21.   Tanvetyanon T, Bepler G. Beta-carotene in multivitamins and the possible risk of lung cancer among smokers versus former smokers: a meta-analysis and evaluation of national brands. *Cancer.* Jul 1 2008;113(1):150-157.

22.   Bjelakovic G, Nagorni A, Nikolova D, Simonetti RG, Bjelakovic M, Gluud C. Meta-analysis: antioxidant supplements for primary and secondary prevention of colorectal adenoma. *Alimentary Pharmacology & Therapeutics.* Jul 15 2006;24(2):281-291.

23.   Bjelakovic G, Nikolova D, Simonetti RG, Gluud C. Systematic review: primary and secondary prevention of gastrointestinal cancers with antioxidant supplements. *Alimentary Pharmacology & Therapeutics.* Sep 15 2008;28(6):689-703.

24. Jiang L, Yang K-h, Tian J-h, et al. Efficacy of antioxidant vitamins and selenium supplement in prostate cancer prevention: a meta-analysis of randomized controlled trials. *Nutrition & Cancer.* Aug 2010;62(6):719-727.

25. Virtamo J, Pietinen P, Huttunen JK, et al. Incidence of cancer and mortality following alpha-tocopherol and beta-carotene supplementation: a postintervention follow-up. *JAMA.* Jul 23 2003;290(4):476-485.

26. Goodman GE, Thornquist MD, Balmes J, et al. The Beta-Carotene and Retinol Efficacy Trial: Incidence of lung cancer and cardiovascular disease mortality during 6-year follow-up after stopping Î²-carotene and retinol supplements. *Journal of the National Cancer Institute.* 2004;96(23):1743-1750.

27. The effect of vitamin E and beta carotene on the incidence of lung cancer and other cancers in male smokers. The Alpha-Tocopherol, Beta Carotene Cancer Prevention Study Group. *New England Journal of Medicine.* Apr 14 1994;330(15):1029-1035.

28. Omenn GS, Goodman GE, Thornquist MD, et al. Effects of a combination of beta carotene and vitamin A on lung cancer and cardiovascular disease. *New England Journal of Medicine.* May 2 1996;334(18):1150-1155.

29. Hennekens CH, Buring JE, Manson JE, et al. Lack of effect of long-term supplementation with beta carotene on the incidence of malignant neoplasms and cardiovascular disease. *New England Journal of Medicine.* May 2 1996;334(18):1145-1149.

30. Lee IM, Cook NR, Manson JE, Buring JE, Hennekens CH. Beta-carotene supplementation and incidence of cancer and cardiovascular disease: the Women's Health Study. *Journal of the National Cancer Institute.* Dec 15 1999;91(24):2102-2106.

31. Lippman SM, Klein EA, Goodman PJ, et al. Effect of selenium and vitamin E on risk of prostate cancer and other cancers: the Selenium and Vitamin E Cancer Prevention Trial (SELECT). *JAMA.* Jan 7 2009;301(1):39-51.

32. Klein EA, Thompson IM, Jr., Tangen CM, et al. Vitamin E and the risk of prostate cancer: the Selenium and Vitamin E Cancer Prevention Trial (SELECT). *JAMA.* Oct 12 2011;306(14):1549-1556.

33. Leppala JM, Virtamo J, Fogelholm R, et al. Controlled trial of alpha-tocopherol and beta-carotene supplements on stroke incidence and mortality in male smokers. *Arteriosclerosis, Thrombosis & Vascular Biology.* Jan 2000;20(1):230-235.

34. Marchioli R, Levantesi G, Macchia A, et al. Vitamin E increases the risk of developing heart failure after myocardial infarction: Results from the GISSI-Prevenzione trial. *Journal of Cardiovascular Medicine.* May 2006;7(5):347-350.

35. Lonn E, Bosch J, Yusuf S, et al. Effects of long-term vitamin E supplementation on cardiovascular events and cancer: a randomized controlled trial. *JAMA.* Mar 16 2005;293(11):1338-1347.

36.   Burr ML, Ashfield-Watt PAL, Dunstan FDJ, et al. Lack of benefit of dietary advice to men with angina: results of a controlled trial. *European Journal of Clinical Nutrition.* Feb 2003;57(2):193-200.

37.   Bairati I, Roy L, Meyer F. Double-blind, randomized, controlled trial of fish oil supplements in prevention of recurrence of stenosis after coronary angioplasty. *Circulation.* Mar 1992;85(3):950-956.

38.   Leaf A, Jorgensen MB, Jacobs AK, et al. Do fish oils prevent restenosis after coronary angioplasty? *Circulation.* Nov 1994;90(5):2248-2257.

39.   Kaul U, Sanghvi S, Bahl VK, Dev V, Wasir HS. Fish oil supplements for prevention of restenosis after coronary angioplasty. *International Journal of Cardiology.* Apr 1992;35(1):87-93.

40.   Kowey PR, Reiffel JA, Ellenbogen KA, Naccarelli GV, Pratt CM. Efficacy and safety of prescription omega-3 fatty acids for the prevention of recurrent symptomatic atrial fibrillation: a randomized controlled trial. *JAMA.* Dec 1 2010;304(21):2363-2372.

41.   Graat JM, Schouten EG, Kok FJ. Effect of daily vitamin E and multivitamin-mineral supplementation on acute respiratory tract infections in elderly persons: a randomized controlled trial. *JAMA.* Aug 14 2002;288(6):715-721.

42.   Johnson AR, Munoz A, Gottlieb JL, Jarrard DF. High dose zinc increases hospital admissions due to genitourinary complications. *Journal of Urology.* Vol 1772007:639-643.

43.   Tardif JC, Cote G, Lesperance J, et al. Probucol and multivitamins in the prevention of restenosis after coronary angioplasty. Multivitamins and Probucol Study Group. *New England Journal of Medicine.* Aug 7 1997;337(6):365-372.

44.   Shao A, Hathcock JN. Risk assessment for the carotenoids lutein and lycopene. *Regulatory Toxicology & Pharmacology.* Aug 2006;45(3):289-298.

45.   Granado F, Olmedilla B, Gil-Martinez E, Blanco I. Lutein ester in serum after lutein supplementation in human subjects. *British Journal of Nutrition.* Nov 1998;80(5):445-449.

46.   Olmedilla B, Granado F, Southon S, et al. A European multicentre, placebo-controlled supplementation study with alpha-tocopherol, carotene-rich palm oil, lutein or lycopene: analysis of serum responses. *Clinical Science.* Apr 2002;102(4):447-456.

47.   Leng GC, Lee AJ, Fowkes FG, et al. Randomized controlled trial of gamma-linolenic acid and eicosapentaenoic acid in peripheral arterial disease. *Clinical Nutrition.* Dec 1998;17(6):265-271.

48.   Edited by Holz FG, Spaide RF. *Medical Retina - Essentials in Ophthalmology.* Berlin Heidelberg New York: Springer; 2007.

PENDIX A. SEARCH STRATEGY

MEDLINE® and Ovid OLDMEDLINE® 1947 to February Week 1 2011 -- Date Searched 2011/02/15 - QUESTION 1

Concept	Search String	N
Age-related macular degeneration	Exp macular degeneration/ OR geographic atrophy/ OR macular edema/ OR wet macular degeneration/ OR macular degeneration.mp OR AMD.mp OR ((moderate OR intermediate) ADJ5 (macular degeneration OR AMD OR maculopathS OR macular dystrophS)).mp OR (age ADJ4 maculopathS).mp OR (age ADJ4 macular).mp OR (retinal ADJ4 degeneration).mp OR macular dystrophy.mp OR Retinal drusen/ OR retinal druseS.mp OR Retinal neovascularization/ OR Retinal Pigment Epithelium/ OR retinal pigment epithelium hyperplasia.mp OR RPE.mp OR retinal pigment epithelium atrophS.mp OR retinal pigment epithelium depigmentation.mp OR geographic atrophy.mp OR Choroidal neovascularization/ OR Choroidal neovascularization.mp OR AREDS stage 1.mp OR AREDS stage 3.mp OR subjacent retinal pigmentation epithelium.mp OR choriocapillaris.mp OR lipofuscin.mp OR neovascular AMD.mp OR CNV.mp OR macular pigment optical density.mp OR MPOD.mp OR (age ADJ1 related ADJ1 eye ADJ1 disease ADJ1 study).mp OR Pigment epithelium of eye/ OR Macula Lutea/ OR fovea centralis/ OR Retinal detachment/	57,272
Nutritional supplements, carotenoids, antioxidants, omega 3 fatty acids	Dietary supplements/ OR (dietary ADJ1 supplementS).mp OR (nutritional ADJ1 supplementS).mp OR Vitamins/ OR Carotenoids/ OR carotenoidS.mp OR zeaxanthin.mp OR Lutein/ OR lutein.mp OR Beta carotene/ OR beta-carotene.mp OR beta carotene.mp OR Antioxidants/ OR antioxidantS.mp OR Zinc/ OR zinc.mp OR Vitamin E/ OR (vitamin ADJ1 E).mp OR Ascorbic acid/ OR (vitamin ADJ1 C).mp OR Fatty Acids, Omega-3/ OR omega 3 fatty acids.mp OR alpha-Linolenic Acid/ OR alpha linolenic acid.mp OR Docosahexaenoic Acids/ OR Docosahexaenoic acid.mp OR Eicosapentaenoic Acid/ OR Eicosapentaenoic acid.mp OR tocopherols.mp	268,101
Cochrane Reviews Clinical Hedge	(randomized controlled trial OR controlled clinical trial OR meta-analysis).pt OR controlled clinical trial OR meta-analysis).pt OR randomized.ab OR placebo.ab OR drug therapy.fs OR randomly.ab OR trial.ab OR groups.ab OR (systematic ADJ1 review).mp	2,611,405
Q1:	1 AND 2 AND 3	**523**

BASE -- Date Searched 2011/03/17 - QUESTION 1

Concept	Search String	N
Age-related macular degeneration	'retina macula age related degeneration'/exp OR 'retina macula degeneration'/exp OR 'retina macula edema'/exp OR 'drusen'/exp OR 'retina neovascularization'/exp OR 'pigment epithelium'/exp OR 'subretinal neovascularization'/exp OR 'retina macula lutea'/exp OR 'retina fovea'/exp OR 'retina detachment'/exp OR 'macular degeneration'/de OR 'macular degeneration' OR 'geographic atrophy' OR 'macular edema'/de OR 'macular edema' OR 'wet macular degeneration' OR 'amd'/de OR amd OR (moderate OR intermediate) NEAR/5 ('macular degeneration' OR amd OR maculopat* OR 'macular dystrophy') OR age NEAR/4 maculopath* OR age NEAR/4 macular OR retinal NEAR/4 degenerat* OR 'macular dystrophy'/de OR 'macular dystrophy' OR rpe OR 'retinal pigment epithelium atrophy' OR 'retinal pigment epithelium depigmentation' OR 'areds stage 1' OR 'areds stage 3' OR 'subjacent retinal pigmentation epithelium' OR 'choriocapillaris'/de OR choriocapillaris OR 'lipofuscin'/de OR lipofuscin OR 'neovascular amd' OR cnv OR 'macular pigment optical density' OR mpod AND [embase]/lim *search also required that the term be a major focus of the article	46,770
Nutritional supplements, carotenoids, antioxidants, omega 3 fatty acids	'diet supplementation'/exp OR 'vitamin'/exp OR 'carotenoid'/exp OR 'xanthophyll'/exp OR 'beta carotene'/exp OR 'antioxidant'/exp OR 'zinc'/exp OR 'alpha tocopherol'/exp OR 'ascorbic acid'/exp OR 'omega 3 fatty acid'/exp OR 'linolenic acid'/exp OR 'docosahexaenoic acid'/exp OR 'icosapentaenoic acid'/exp OR 'tocopherol'/exp OR 'zeaxanthin'/exp	538,080

Cochrane Reviews Clinical Hedge	'randomized controlled trial'/exp OR 'controlled clinical trial'/exp OR 'meta analysis'/exp OR 'systematic review'/exp	380,031
	* Also searched as keyword and major focus of article	
Q1:	1 AND 2 AND 3	146

HRANE (Cochrane Database of Systematic Reviews; Database of Abstracts of Reviews of Effects; Cochrane Central Register of Controlled Trials)
te Searched 2011/03/28 - QUESTION 1

Concept	Search String	N
Age-related macular degeneration	"macular degeneration" OR "geographic atroph*" OR "macular edema" OR AMD "macular dystroph*" OR "Retinal druse*" OR "Retinal neovascularization" OR "Retinal Pigment Epithelium" OR RPE OR "Choroidal neovascularization" OR AREDS OR choriocapillaris OR lipofuscin OR "neovascular AMD" OR CNV OR "macular pigment optical density" OR MPOD OR "Macula Lutea" OR "fovea centralis" OR "Retinal detachment" (Title, Abstracts, or Keywords search)	28
Nutritional supplements, carotenoids, antioxidants, omega 3 fatty acids	Supplement* OR vitamin* OR carotenoid* OR xanthophyll OR beta carotene* OR antioxidant* OR zinc OR tocopherol* OR "ascorbic acid" OR "omega 3 fatty acid*" OR linolenic OR docosahexaenoic OR icosapentaenoic OR zeaxanthin (Title, Abstracts, or Keywords search)	530
Q1:	1 AND 2	3

PUS -- Date Searched 2011/03/28 - QUESTION 1

Concept	Search String	N
Age-related macular degeneration	macular degeneration OR geographic atroph* OR macular edema OR AMD macular dystroph* OR Retinal druse* OR Retinal neovascularization OR Retinal Pigment Epithelium OR RPE OR choroidal neovascularization OR AREDS OR choriocapillaris OR lipofuscin OR neovascular AMD OR CNV OR macular pigment optical density OR MPOD OR Macula Lutea OR fovea centralis OR Retinal detachment (Title, Abstracts, or Keywords search)	73,074
Nutritional supplements, carotenoids, antioxidants, omega 3 fatty acids	Supplement* OR vitamin* OR carotenoid* OR xanthophyll OR beta carotene* OR antioxidant* OR zinc OR tocopherol* OR "ascorbic acid" OR "omega 3 fatty acid*" OR linolenic OR docosahexaenoic OR icosapentaenoic OR zeaxanthin (Keywords search)	4,296
Q1:	1 AND 2	73

erence Papers Index -- Date Searched 2011/03/28 - QUESTION 1

Concept	Search String	N
Age-related macular degeneration	macular degeneration OR geographic atroph* OR macular edema OR AMD macular dystroph* OR Retinal druse* OR Retinal neovascularization OR Retinal Pigment Epithelium OR RPE OR choroidal neovascularization OR AREDS OR choriocapillaris OR lipofuscin OR neovascular AMD OR CNV OR macular pigment optical density OR MPOD OR Macula Lutea OR fovea centralis OR Retinal detachment (Keywords search)	3,832
Nutritional supplements, carotenoids, antioxidants, omega 3 fatty acids	Supplement* OR vitamin* OR carotenoid* OR xanthophyll OR beta carotene* OR antioxidant* OR zinc OR tocopherol* OR "ascorbic acid" OR "omega 3 fatty acid*" OR linolenic OR docosahexaenoic OR icosapentaenoic OR zeaxanthin (Keywords search)	22,207
Q1:	1 AND 2	68

MEDLINE® and Ovid OLDMEDLINE® 1947 to February Week 4 2011 -- Date Searched 2011/02/15 - QUESTION 2 SEARCH

Concept	Search String	N
Population	Aging/ OR aging.mp. OR ageing.mp. OR Aged/ OR aged.mp. OR "Aged, 80 and over"/ OR frail elderly/ OR Middle aged/ OR middle aged.mp. OR elderS.mp. OR seniorS.mp. OR geriatricS.mp. OR geriatric/ OR age-related.mp. OR (age adj1 related).mp.	3,562,146
Zeaxanthin, lutein, beta-carotene, zinc, vitamin e, vitamin c, alpha linolenic acid, DHA, EPA	zeaxanthin.mp OR Lutein/ OR lutein.mp OR Beta carotene/ OR beta-carotene.mp OR beta carotene.mp OR Zinc/ OR zinc. mp OR Vitamin E/ OR (vitamin ADJ1 E).mp OR tocopherols.mp OR Ascorbic acid/ OR (vitamin ADJ1 C).mp OR alpha-Linolenic Acid/ OR alpha linolenic acid.mp OR Docosahexaenoic Acids/ OR Docosahexaenoic acid.mp OR Eicosapentaenoic Acid/ OR Eicosapentaenoic acid.mp	160,101
Cochrane Reviews Clinical Hedge	(randomized controlled trial OR controlled clinical trial OR meta-analysis).pt OR randomized.ab OR placebo.ab OR drug therapy.fs OR randomly.ab OR trial.ab OR groups.ab OR (systematic ADJ1 review).mp	2,656,105
Harms	unsafe.mp OR safety.mp OR harm.mp OR harms.mp OR complications.mp OR poisonS.mp OR riskS.mp OR AE.fs OR MO.fs OR PO.fs OR TO.fs OR CT.fs OR side-effectS.mp OR (undesirable ADJ1 effectS).mp OR (treatment ADJ1 emergent).mp OR tolerabS.mp OR toxicS.mp OR adrs.mp OR (adverse ADJ2 (effect or effects or reaction or reactions or event or events or outcome or outcomes)).mp	3,492,667
Q2:	1 AND 2 AND 3 AND 4	**3,514**
Population, dietary supplements, study methods, and harms		

ase -- Date Searched 2011/03/17 - QUESTION 2

Concept	Search String	N
Population	'aged'/mj OR 'frail elderly'/mj OR 'elderly'/mj OR 'very elderly'/mj OR 'aged hospital patient'/mj OR 'middle aged'/mj OR senior* OR geriatric* OR 'age near/1 related' AND [embase]/lim	154,441
Zeaxanthin, lutein, beta-carotene, zinc, vitamin e, vitamin c, alpha linolenic acid, DHA, EPA	'diet supplementation'/mj OR 'carotenoid'/mj OR 'xanthophyll'/mj OR 'beta carotene'/mj OR 'antioxidant'/mj OR 'zinc'/mj OR 'alpha tocopherol'/mj OR 'ascorbic acid'/mj OR 'omega 3 fatty acid'/mj OR 'linolenic acid'/mj OR 'docosahexaenoic acid'/mj OR 'icosapentaenoic acid'/mj OR 'tocopherol'/mj OR 'zeaxanthin'/mj AND [embase]/lim	98,250
Cochrane Reviews Clinical Hedge	'randomized controlled trial'/mj OR 'randomized controlled trial'/de OR 'randomized controlled clinical trial'/mj OR 'controlled clinical trial'/de OR 'controlled clinical trial'/mj OR 'meta analysis'/mj OR 'meta analysis'/de OR 'meta analysis' OR 'systematic review'/mj OR 'systematic review'/de OR 'systematic review' AND [embase]/lim

*also searched as keyword and main topic of article | 380,031 |
| Harms | 'adverse drug reaction'/mj OR 'adverse drug reaction' OR 'drug induced disease' OR 'drug induced disease'/mj OR 'complication'/mj OR 'complication' OR 'intoxication'/mj OR 'intoxication' OR 'toxicity'/mj OR 'toxicity' OR 'drug hypersensitivity'/mj OR 'drug hypersensitivity' OR unsafe OR 'safety'/mj OR safety OR harm OR harms OR complication* OR poison* OR risk* OR undesirable NEAR/1 effect OR treatment NEAR/1 emergent OR tolerab* OR toxic* OR adrs OR adverse NEAR/2 (effect OR effects OR reaction OR reactions OR event OR events OR outcome OR outcomes) AND [embase]/lim | 3,965,190 |

Q2:	1 AND 2 AND 3 AND 4	108
Population, dietary supplements, study methods, and harms		

PUS -- Date Searched 2011/03/17 - QUESTION 2

Concept	Search String	N
Population	aged OR elderly OR "middle aged" OR senior* OR geriatric* OR "age related" in TITLE-ABS-KEY	3,178,852
Zeaxanthin, lutein, beta-carotene, zinc, vitamin e, vitamin c, alpha linolenic acid, DHA, EPA	zeaxanthin OR lutein OR "Beta carotene" OR zinc OR "Vitamin E" OR tocopherol* OR "Ascorbic acid" OR "vitamin C" OR alpha-linolenic OR docosahexaenoic OR eicosapentaenoic in TITLE-ABS-KEY-AUTH	447,672
Cochrane Reviews Clinical Hedge	"randomized controlled trial*" OR "controlled clinical trial*" OR "meta analysis" OR "systematic review*" TITLE-ABS-KEY-AUTH	529,484
Harms	"adverse drug reaction*" OR "adverse reaction*" OR complication* OR toxic* OR poison* OR harm* OR unsafe OR tolerab* OR adverse outcome* OR adverse event* OR adverse effect* TITLE-ABS-KEY-AUTH	252,917
Q2:	1 AND 2 AND 3 AND 4	309
Population, dietary supplements, study methods, and harms		

rane Library (Cochrane Database of Systematic Reviews; Database of Abstracts of Reviews of Effects; Cochrane Central Register of Controlled Trials) -- Searched 2011/03/25 - QUESTION 2

Concept	Search String	N
Population	aged OR elderly OR "middle aged" OR senior* OR geriatric* OR "age related" (Title, Abstracts or Keywords search)	1,238
Zeaxanthin, lutein, beta-carotene, zinc, vitamin e, vitamin c, alpha linolenic acid, DHA, EPA	zeaxanthin OR lutein OR "Beta carotene" OR zinc OR "Vitamin E" OR tocopherol* OR "Ascorbic acid" OR "vitamin C" OR alpha-linolenic OR docosahexaenoic OR eicosapentaenoic (Title, Abstracts or Keywords search)	79
Harms	reaction* OR complication* OR toxic* OR poison* OR harm* OR unsafe OR safety OR tolerab* OR adverse (Title, Abstracts or Keywords search)	4,283
Q2:	1 AND 2 AND 3	23
Population, dietary supplements, study methods, and harms		

erence Papers Index -- Date Searched 2011/03/25 - QUESTION 2

Concept	Search String	N
Population	aged OR elderly OR "middle aged" OR senior* OR geriatric* OR "age related" (Keyword search)	21,302

Zeaxanthin, lutein, beta-carotene, zinc, vitamin e, vitamin c, alpha linolenic acid, DHA, EPA	zeaxanthin OR lutein OR "Beta carotene" OR zinc OR "Vitamin E" OR tocopherol* OR "Ascorbic acid" OR "vitamin C" OR "omega 3 fatty acid*" OR alpha-linolenic OR docosahexaenoic OR eicosapentaenoic (Keyword search)	9,376
Harms	reaction* OR complication* OR toxic* OR poison* OR harm* OR unsafe OR safety OR tolerab* OR adverse (Keyword search)	98,395
Q2:	1 AND 2 AND 3	1
Population, dietary supplements, study methods, and harms		

APPENDIX B. INCLUSION/EXCLUSION CRITERIA

1. Is the full text of the article in English?
   Yes..Proceed to #2
   No...Code **X1**. STOP

2. Is the article a controlled clinical trial or a systematic review/meta-analysis of controlled trials comparing the effects of supplemental/non-dietary carotenoids, antioxidants, or omega-3 fatty acids (alone or in combination) with usual care or placebo?
   Yes..Proceed to #3
   No ....Code **X2**. Go to #6

3. Does the population include adults with age-related macular degeneration?
   Yes..Proceed to #4
   No..Proceed to #5

4. Does the study report outcomes that include vision loss, quality of life, functional status, or adverse effects of treatment?
   Yes... Code **I4**. STOP
   No..Code **X4**. Go to #6

5. Does the study report the adverse effects of treatment in a population of ≥100 adults without age-related macular degeneration who were observed for >24 weeks?
   Yes... Code **I5**. STOP
   No...Code **X5**. Proceed to #6

6. Is the article potentially useful for background, discussion, or reference-mining?
   Yes... Add Code **B**. STOP
   No.. STOP

PICOTS
Patients: KQ1: Adults with age-related macular degeneration
           KQ2: Adults, exclude patients with severe chronic illnesses such as end-stage liver disease, ESRD, severe COPD, metastatic cancer, ALS, severe heart failure

Interventions: Carotenoids – zeaxanthin, lutein, beta-carotene
                 Antioxidants – zinc, vitamin e, vitamin c
                 Omega-3 fatty acids – alpha linolenic acid (C18:3n-3), docosahexaenoic acid (DHA; C22:6n-3), eicosapentaenoic acid (EPA; C20:5n-3)

Comparators: Placebo, usual care (usual diet)

Outcomes: Vision loss
Visual impairment in the best eye defined as: ≤ 20/60 by Snellen acuity; or ≤ 6/18 metric acuity; or doubling of the visual angle (e.g. 20/50 to 20/100); or ≥ three lines of loss; or ≥ 15 letters lost; or progression to advanced disease (either geographic atrophy or wet macular degeneration); quality of life; functional status.

PENDIX C. ASSESSMENT OF METHODOLOGIC QUALITY AND RISK OF BIAS IN RANDOMIZED NTROLLED TRIALS OF ORAL SUPPLEMENTS FOR AGE-RELATED MACULAR DEGENERATION

udy	Allocation sequence adequately generated	Allocation adequately concealed	Blinding of participants, personnel and outcome assessors	Incomplete outcome data adequately addressed	Absence of selective outcome reporting	Free of other sources of bias	Overall risk of bias	Funding source
EDS, 01[10]	Yes; randomization by treatment center then patients assigned with probability to 1/4 to each group.	Yes	Yes; all meds and placebo were coded and concealed from subjects and examiners…codes were kept only in the coordinating center.	Yes; participants were dropped if not photographed or proper visual acuity measurements were not obtained…these dropped subjects were "evenly distributed across the groups". Only 2.4% of subjects were lost to follow-up (missed at least 2 consecutive visits).	Yes; each stated outcome measure was reported in addition to adverse events.	Yes	Low	NIH; Bausch & Lomb Inc.
2005[16]	Yes; computer generated randomization sequence.	Yes; staff and subjects were masked.	Yes; all meds and placebos were masked from both subjects and investigators.	Yes; ITT analysis was done; 5/106 failed to complete study and details were reported of each.	Yes; outcomes were reported as indicated.	Yes	Low	Funding NR
some, 88[11]	Yes	Yes	Yes	Unclear	Yes	Yes	Low	Research Fund Department of Veterinary Science, Utah State University
some, 08[14]	Yes; randomized with 50% likeli-hood scheme (Yes; 50% likeli-hood scheme).	Yes; study coor-dinator provided supplements but did not complete data collection.	Yes; supplements identical in appearance.	Unclear; did not include data from subjects who dropped out or died.	Yes	Yes	Low	Retinal Disease Research Foundation
1996[15]	Yes	Yes	Yes	Unclear: 12 of 71 rate of attrition, but no data provided for those patients, including treatment assignment.	Yes	Yes; 17% loss to follow-up, unclear treatment assignment.	Low	Twin Laboratories, Inc.; Eye Communications, Inc.; Stereo Optical, Inc; Illinois College of Optometry; Pacific University College of Optometry; Ezell Foundation, American Academy of Optometry
2004[12]	Yes; random card.	Yes	Yes	Yes	Yes	Yes	Low	DVA Medical Center, North Chicago; Kemin Foods, Vitacost.com; Nutraceutical Sciences Institute; Great Smokies Diagnostic Laboratory
1996[13]	Unclear; random-ization method not described.	Yes	Yes	Yes	Yes	Yes	Low	Austrian Foundation for the Propagation of Scientific Research

ENDIX D. PEER REVIEW COMMENTS AND RESPONSES

wer	Comment	Response
ion 1: Are the objectives, scope, and methods for this review clearly described?		
	It is clear in the Methods section that your literature focuses on patients with ARMD, although in the Background of the Executive Summary and the Introduction, it is noted that "observational studies suggest that people with dietary intakes higher in various nutritional supplements have a lower risk of developing AMD". Yet there is no mention of the data indicating that nutritional supplements may have a role in preventing ARMD. Since the data evaluating prevention of ARMD is not even addressed, perhaps a statement recognizing that prevention data exists, but is outside the realm of this report would be beneficial.	The comment in the background was modified to clarify our purpose. The statement identifies the reason large supplementation trials were initiated to investigate the role of dietary supplements in AMD prevention. We note there is a large body of observational data suggesting dietary antioxidants, carotenoids and/or fish oils may be beneficial. This data is not reviewed here because of the risk of uncontrolled confounding and recall bias in observational cohort studies.
3	Yes; Specific aims of study and methods are clearly described and are appropriate.	Noted, thank you.
4	Yes; Thorough and excellent review	Noted, thank you.
ion 2: Is there any indication of bias in our synthesis of the evidence?		
4	Yes... and this is clearly stated at the very beginning of the report (It should also be stated in the conclusion) On page 3, the authors reject 298 of 335 (89 %) full-text scientific articles (1000+ authors) not meeting the inclusion criteria of EBM; 2) Throughout the entire report, the term "Functional" is used rather than the more precise term "Snellen Visual Acuity"; 3) Key Question 1: Limiting most all discussions of carotenoids to primarily a B carotene and all antioxidants to 1 form of the 8 isomers of vitamin E (i.e. alpha tocopherol) is an oversimplification of nature and known science, (despite the fact that another government agency (NEI / NIH) made this decision to persist in using the same 1990s nutritional components in the "new" AREDS II study). Given the relative lack of information ??? about the effects of xanthophylls, carotenoids and omega III fatty acids, future trials should be considered to assess the effects of these supplements in AMD patients". The term "information" should be replaced with "EBM" to be consistent. There are 1000's of scientific articles concerning n3 fatty acids, and dozens concerning the salutary benefit for AMD patients and people worried about not getting it. I know of only a single negative omega III – AMD study.	The inclusion and exclusion criteria were pre-specified before we undertook the review. The outcomes of interest and interventions of interest were determined based on discussion with a Technical Expert Panel.

In the methods section, we defined functional vision loss in a variety of ways using both Snellen and non-Snellen methods.

Given the problems inherent with observational data, we included only RCTs and only found one RCT of omega IIIs evaluating the outcomes of interest |
2	No.	Noted, thank you.
3	There is no evidence of bias. English only studies were examined, but this is appropriate for age-related macular degeneration as Caucasians are most frequently affected and relevant studies are in English. Appropriate steps were taken to review appropriate studies in a systemic manor with accepted evaluation techniques.	Noted, thank you.
4	No.	Noted, thank you.
ion 3: Are there any published or unpublished studies that we may have overlooked?		
1	The report does not list the 298 rejected studies.	Although we do not list excluded studies in our report, we can provide a list of excluded studies and reasons for exclusion separately upon request.

40

ewer	Comment	Response
1	Lintje Ho, MD et al The Rotterdam Study Reducing the Genetic Risk of AMD with Dietary Antioxidants, Zinc and w3 fatty acids *Arch Ophthalmol. 2011; 129 (6):758-66* (High dietary intake of nutrients with antioxidant properties reduces the risk of early AMD in those at high genetic risk. Therefore, clinicians should provide dietary advice to young susceptible individuals to postpone or prevent the vision-disturbing consequences of AMD).	Thank you for suggesting this study. Our scope and inclusion criteria would exclude this study because the focus of the review is on supplemental rather than dietary intake of antioxidants.
1	*Christen GS et al,* The Women's Health Study - Dietary w3 Fatty Acid and Fish Intake and Incident AMD in Women *Arch Ophthalmol. 2011; 129 (7):921-9* (These prospective data from a large cohort of female health professionals without a diagnosis of AMD at baseline indicate that regular consumption of DHAA and EPA and fish was associated with a significantly decreased risk of incident AMD and may be of benefit in primary prevention of AMD).	Our scope and inclusion criteria would exclude this study as well because the focus of the review is on supplemental rather than dietary intake of antioxidants.
2	Under **Other Adverse Effects,** *Yellowing of the skin:* it only notes that beta-carotene is associated with yellowing of the skin. This effect is also noted with lutein. See ref: Regul Toxicol Pharmacol 2006; 45: 289-298.	We have added this suggested narrative review and references for the two trials it cites regarding lutein supplementation and carotenodermia.
3	No.	Noted, thank you.
4	Not that I am aware.	Noted, thank you.
tion 4: Please write additional suggestions or comments below. If applicable, please indicate the page and line numbers from the draft report.		
4	The 1862 legal term Snellen Visual Acuity throughout the report is used to define both "function" and "stage of disease". However, foveal vision in humans is, more often than not, highly conserved until the patho-physiology of AMD has run its course. It is therefore a poor term to use to describe both functional vision and the stage of disease in either dry or wet AMD. Thus the EBM model adopted within this report is in complete opposition to biology and the patient-doctor encounter. It contradicts the results of both the LAST study 2004 and our recently published ZVF study (FDA #78,973). In both studies patients had better than 20/32 visual acuity yet poor contrast sensitivity and glare recovery...i.e. they had visual disability. If we use an AREDS deterministic legal definition of 15 letter Snellen improvement, your report is correct to assume that ours were negative studies by definition.	The outcomes of interest were determined after discussion with a group of technical experts who felt functional vision loss as we've defined it was the appropriate outcome to evaluate for the systematic review. Evaluation of these more proximal outcome metrics is outside the scope of our review.

wer	Comment	Response
	In this report, it was stated not once but twice that AMD changes occur slowly over time. I agree, but only if one is younger than 85 – then the changes will occur very quickly. Furthermore, such aged individuals are the fastest growing demographic in the United States. There are 10x the number of patients with AMD between age 85 and 95 compared to ages 75 – 85 (and not double). We are wasting time.	We agree and have added the suggested text to the Discussion section.
	Excellent report. Thank you for taking the time to develop this document. One suggestion would be to provide references to the studies noted in the Executive Summary Table on page 6.	We have added the study references to the summary table in the Conclusions of the main report, as suggested. We generally do not include citations in the Executive Summary.
	Under **Study Selection**, it is noted that only those studies with at least 24 weeks of follow-up and sample size of 100 were included, but some of the data is not consistent with that statement. For example, the Newsome, 2008 trial only contained 74 participants.	We have clarified the methods to specify that we did not limit the sample size or duration of treatment of RCTs to answer the question of efficacy. Sample size of 100 or more pertained to included studies of adverse effects.
	EDRTS is used throughout the document. It should be ETDRS for Early Treatment Diabetic Retinopathy Study	Thank you for this correction. We have changed "EDTRS" to "ETDRS" throughout the document.
	The reviewers did an excellent job of identifying the categories of AMD and incorporating the relative susceptibility as part of their evaluation. For example, studies evaluating patients with Category 1 and 2 AMD are not likely to find a benefit to supplementation given the gradual nature of the disease process as well as the lack of vision loss in these categories. This finding is of crucial importance in determining which patients may benefit from supplementation that does carry some risk.	Noted, thank you.
	I feel the comment on page 4 that there are not effective therapies is out of sequence. I am not sure this is born out in the grade 3 and 4 AMD patients with the supplements. Overall the paper is correct; clinicians refer to the AREDS trial as an indication of the use of supplements as the only valid trial. As you noted there is additional AREDS2 looking at adding carotenoids in progress. Also, there is a "smokers" AREDS without the antioxidants that may reduce the risk of lung cancer? I think the part that remains difficult is the assessment of the risk. If there were even marginal benefit and no risk then the treatment strategy is clear. I think you have addressed this in as much detail as is currently available	We have deleted the first sentence to improve clarity. We added text to the Discussion section regarding the amendment to the AREDS study in which smokers were offered a chance to change their randomization of treatment supplements to either zinc alone (without the antioxidants) or placebo.
	Page 3, 4th paragraph: In the AREDS study- please specify AREDS 1 and list the formula components.	Done.
	Page 4 and through the document: please define "former" smoker if that information is given in the reviewed studies.	We have added definitions for "former" smoker, as suggested.
	Page 5, 1st paragraph: "Higher doses of vit E have been associated with increased mortality and congestive heart failure among those with high baseline risk". High baseline risk needs to be defined. What constitutes high baseline risk? Also, "carotenoids such as beta-carotene have been associated with an increased risk of lung cancer among smokers. The absolute risk of harm is low." How low is low? please clarify here.	We have added the estimated magnitude of increased risk for each outcome in this paragraph.

ewer	Comment	Response
	Page 6-7: executive summary table. In the Comment Column, it would be nice to have the actual doses listed to help understand what authors mean by High-dose vit E, beta-carotene, etc. Also 'high risk patients" needs to be clarified.	Thank you for this suggestion. We have added the dose range to the Summary Table to better characterize the high-dose and low-dose studies. We have also added a footnote in Table 1 to specify the definition of high vs low risk AMD used in Stur, 1996.
	Page 9, 1 paragraph, 1 line: The natural history of AMD has not been shown definitely to have been altered by any treatment modality. The authors should specify that they are specifically looking at the *nonexudative* AMD.	Thank you for this suggestion, however, we have decided to delete this sentence to improve clarity in response to another comment.
	Page 10, under Patients: Adults with age-related macular degeneration - please specify *nonexudative* age-related macular degeneration is being studied here.	Done.
	Outcomes: It would be nice to point out here that a 3-line change in visual acuity (i.e. +/- 15 letters) using the ETDRS chart is equivalent to a doubling or halving of the visual angle regardless of the baseline visual acuity measurement.	We have added the suggested text to the list of outcomes in the Methods section.
	Page 11, Fig 1. Adult outpatients with (NON-EXUDATIVE- please add) age-related macular degeneration	Done.
	Page 14, 2nd paragraph: Please add a reference at the end of the sentence that talks about the GRADE working group.	Citation added.
	Page 18, 2nd paragraph: "In analysis limited to only those with Category 3 or 4 AMD, a reduction in functional visual loss was noted with either supplement alone or in combination." should be clarified by specifying how much improvement was detected with either and with the combination.	Thank you for this suggestion. We have revised the paragraph accordingly.
	The last sentence" No baseline characteristic differences were noted between the Category 2, 3, or 4 participants." is confusing, since these categories of participants are inherently different from each other. Not sure what the sentence is saying. Please clarify.	We have clarified this sentence to read: "No significant differences in demographics, socioeconomic status, smoking status, or comorbidities were noted between the Category 2, 3 or 4 participants."
	Page 20-22: Table 1. The 4th-6th columns list outcomes, however no P-values are listed to make sense of numbers listed. Please include P-values (from articles listed) wherever is possible.	Done.
	Page 23: "Additionally, the treatment arms will evaluate the effects of eliminating beta-carotene for the original AREDS formulation..." should be FROM the original AREDS. Would also be nice to list the ingredients of the AREDS formulation here.	Thank you for this correction. We have specified the ingredients of the original AREDS formulation, as suggested.
	Page 26, under Lung Cancer: please define what was meant by "former smokers". How many years after quitting tobacco?	We have added definitions for "former" smokers, as suggested.

www.ingramcontent.com/pod-product-compliance